Easy as Pie Keto Fasting Guide

Fast and Effective Weight Loss with Intermittent Fasting +
Keto Diet (A Beginner Friendly Guide for Women)

By: Susan Katz

TABLE OF CONTENTS

Introduction

So here we are then. You've probably picked up this book after your latest diet has failed. Or perhaps you're simply tired of what you see in the mirror every time you look. You feel sluggish, overweight, and a climb up the stairs gets you huffing and puffing like you're trying to blow someone's house down.

By this time, you've probably tried a few diets and perhaps even saw some fleeting success with some of them. However, you must have then run into what every dieter out there experiences: the plateau. After that initial burst of weight loss, nothing happens, and you remain the same, except you're now working twice as hard, counting your calories the whole way.

Oh yeah, there's the counting calories bit. All of a sudden, food isn't food to you; it's some combination of calories which causes you to think about all the time. Does this put me over my caloric requirement? Can I afford, calorically speaking, to eat this now? Will, I put on more fat if I eat this?

It's safe to say that no matter what your intentions were when you started, they've been completely subverted thanks to the demands your previous diets have placed on you. You started out wanting to look and feel good. Instead, all those diets have now made you feel like you're attempting rocket science while juggling two plates at the same time while riding a bicycle.

I'm here to tell you; all this is coming to a stop right now! That's right! This book has the solution you need, and while it will take some work on your part, I promise you that the results you will see will only spur you on to greater heights. Instead of pouring over all those before/after pictures you see on Instagram, you can now take your own!

Here's my pledge: within four weeks, you will see a leaner, fitter version of yourself in the mirror by following everything laid out in this book.

So How Do I Achieve This?

Losing fat and getting healthy is a simple process that relies on two essential principles: Intermittent fasting (IF) and the Ketogenic diet. You've probably heard of these concepts before but even if you haven't, don't worry. This book is a thirty-day guide to fat loss, and along the way, you will learn all about these concepts and more importantly, how to integrate them into your life successfully.

You see, a lot of diets prescribe something without taking your lifestyle into account. Then, there's the problem of a lot of diets not suiting women. Women face particular challenges that men do not when it comes to fat loss. For one, it is tougher for women to lose fat as compared to men and secondly, we girls tend to second guess ourselves more than the guys out there.

In this book, I've put together both the concepts, with the science behind them, as well as actionable plans for you to get started immediately. None of what I've written in this book is pie-in-the-sky type thinking - it's real and practical. IF and Keto are the most powerful ways to lose fat and get healthy.

By combining them, you get to access the best of both worlds!

Wait, Why Should I Listen to You Anyway?

That's a good question! After all, who am I to lecture you on how to do things? I don't have a string of letters after my name, and neither am I a sexy Instagram babe. No. What I am is a regular gal who went through what you're going through right now and struggled with the same issues that plague you at this moment.

I've never had a model like physique, despite craving one and trying my damnedest to eat as healthy as possible. It seemed like everything I did had just one effect, and that was to increase the size of my waist and put on fat in areas where people would immediately notice. I struggled with body image issues, and these ran so deep that even today, I occasionally struggle with insecurity as well.

Once I gave birth to my child, this problem only became worse. What with my already low self-esteem and the pregnancy weight gain, I felt a growing sense of dread during what should have been one of the happiest moments of my life. Once my baby was born, though, I had a choice to make. I could either set a bad example and resign myself to something I hated, or be active in showing my child how you're supposed to deal with problems.

I discovered the Keto diet, and initially, it didn't make much sense to me. After all, how does eating fat help you lose fat? I decided to try it anyway since I didn't have much to lose. I saw results immediately and began shedding weight. However, I was still struggling to nail my calorie counts, and it was becoming unsustainable. I could tell the progress I had made would soon vanish, and I would regress because the method I was using was unsustainable.

Then I stumbled upon intermittent fasting. On the surface of it, this seemed like another form of food torture, to be honest. Go hungry for sixteen hours a day? Only eat for eight hours? Then again, what did I have to lose? I plunged heart and soul into it. Well, IF turned out to be the easiest thing I had ever done.

I found that my natural eating pattern, indeed the pattern for most of us, follows what IF prescribes. With a few barely noticeable adjustments, I was able to not only follow my plans but even ditch counting calories! That alone made me jump for joy.

Along the way, I also discovered the additional benefits of becoming healthier, and to this day, I continue to follow what's written in this book. There is no further information you need or something special you have to do to achieve the same results. It's all in here!

So, You're Saying It Works?

Absolutely! Once you follow this diet plan, you will see the fat melt right off your body. That's not an empty promise; it's merely the result of you reconnecting with the way human beings are supposed to eat! IF has several proven health benefits and has been practiced since ancient times (Gunnars, 2017).

IF increases your cellular level inflammation, possibly reverses Type 2 diabetes, lowers your blood sugar and insulin levels, and stimulates autophagy (Gunnars, 2017). Meanwhile, the keto diet is no slouch either. Along with the usual effects such as fat loss and increased energy, the keto diet also helps reverse Type 2 diabetes and is prescribed for many Type 1 diabetes patients as well (Gunnars, 2017).

In addition to this, it helps increase the good cholesterol within you and reduces the bad cholesterol, along with lowering your blood pressure (Gunnars, 2017).

If none of this convinces you, well your body's improved and sexy appearance will. I mean, it works for Beyonce, Nicole Kidman, Hugh Jackman, and Jennifer Lopez, so why wouldn't it work for you?

You will also experience the side effects of becoming healthier as I did. Your skin will look better, your overall appearance will be more pleasing, and your mood will be a lot better, thanks to having energy more often. No more huffing and puffing up the stairs!

A Commitment

Let me repeat this: By following the steps outlined in this book, you will not only become and feel healthier, but you will also have your friends come up to you and ask "What the f*ck have you been doing?!"

You will love the new you that appears in the mirror and will have both mental and physical energy as you go about your day. At first, it will seem counterintuitive, but I will show you proof of this working, in addition to what I've already shown you.

Best of all, I've given you a simple and easy to follow plan born out of my own experiences and the mistakes I made. This book is a practical, step by step plan which you will have no problems implementing in your life, and in a month's time, you will notice visible results!

So stop hating yourself and take action! There's no time like the present - indeed, it is the only time available to us. The steps outlined in this book require discipline, but this isn't some Navy Seal-like determination that's being asked of you. No, everything within this book is easily achievable by you, and you already have everything you need to succeed.

Best off all, it doesn't matter whether you're looking to lose five pounds or a hundred and five pounds, the solution is the same! In fact, the more weight you have to lose, the better this method works! You will be combining two of the most potent fat burning tools out there, and you will inevitably become healthy and achieve what you want.

So let's start then, shall we? Are you ready to change your life? Let's get into it!

CHAPTER 1:

WHY INTERMITTENT FASTING+KETO WORKS BETTER...MUCH BETTER

Some of you will be familiar with intermittent fasting and keto as separate concepts, while some of you won't. This chapter is for the latter group, and I'll talk about how IF as well as the ketogenic diet, impact fat loss and overall health. If you're already familiar with this topic and want to get into the nitty-gritty, please feel free to skip ahead to the chapter you wish to learn about, if not, let's get into it.

Fasting, in some form or another, has existed since ancient times as a method to treat disease as well as manage overall health. While a majority of the ancient techniques prescribed fasting periods of a day or sometimes more, intermittent fasting is a scientifically backed approach that removes the guesswork from the process of fasting.

To understand how the ketogenic diet can incorporate within its framework, we need first to understand what intermittent fasting is all about.

Intermittent Fasting

IF has been a fitness trend for a while now, but unlike most trends, this actually works. When your goal is to burn fat, it is your diet that plays the lion's share of the role in the process. With dieting, restrictions comes a variety of permutations and combinations that you need to take into account, and this often complicates things.

You've probably experienced this already with your last diet. The question of what to eat suddenly became a valid and, in some cases, terrifying experience. As you progressed along with your previous diet, the fear of eating the wrong thing would have intensified. A lot of dieters report such feelings when it comes to any diet regimen.

The easiest way to control what you eat is to do what is easily repeatable. In other words, the less you need to think about something, the easier it is to turn it into a habit. Think about it: Do you have to think about tying your shoelaces? No. It's deeply ingrained in your mind.

Similarly, your aim with dieting should be to simplify it as much as possible so that it is easier to adopt into your lifestyle. That's where IF can help.

Benefits

While fat loss is a natural side effect of intermittent fasting, its health benefits go well beyond just that. Here is a small sample of benefits that IF provides.

Autophagy: Autophagy is the process by which cells clean themselves of harmful protein buildup. Thanks to the fasting portion of IF, cells initiate this process. A study conducted in 2010, which aimed to measure the rate at which Autophagy begins, concluded that the number of vesicles per cell (which is a measure of the autophagous response) increased within twenty-four hours of food restriction (Antunes et al., 2018).

Furthermore, autophagosome characteristics are also detected with an increase in the cell area, perimeter, and other physical changes. After forty-eight hours, these characteristics only increased. The results were validated against standard characteristics observed through electron microscopy methods, and thus, the results were deemed valid.

In other words, the biological markers of Autophagy increased significantly.

Metabolic Rate: Fasting intermittently increases our body's metabolic rate, which in turn causes us to burn more food more efficiently and aids in fat loss, depending on the composition of our diet. A study in 2000, aimed at observing the effect of short-term starvation in lean, healthy men and women, found that energy burned while resting increased significantly from the first to the third day (Zauner et al., 2000).

Also, the concentration of norepinephrine increased as well accompanied by a decrease in serum glucose. Insulin was unaffected throughout. The researchers concluded that the increase in plasma norepinephrine was due to the decline in glucose and was a marker of biological changes upon the initiation of starvation.

Given the increase in energy expenditure, this was an indication that the metabolic rate had increased.

Aside from these benefits, there is also evidence that IF increases the secretion of HGH, or human growth hormone, which helps in muscle building and fat loss, as well as reduces the levels of insulin in the body which makes the fat more accessible to burn (Gunnars, 2017).

Following intermittent fasting, the plan is quite straight forward. There aren't many rules or regulations for you to follow, unlike other diets. However, there are some mental blocks that always trip people up.

So let me first address these bogus claims, and then I'll show you the different methods by which you can implement IF in your life.

Pattern

Let me say this right off the bat: human beings are perfectly capable of functioning without food for long periods of time (Gunnars, 2017). I'm not talking a few hours; I'm talking days. In ancient times, it was common for our ancestors to go without food for days. After all, it's not as if deer and other food simply offered themselves up to be eaten willingly.

Thus, if you're worried about failing to function or concerned about your activity levels dropping, rest assured. Your concerns are legitimate, but your brain is amplifying the doubt within because you're so used to a particular pattern of eating that anything else strikes you as being unnatural. Never mind the fact that fasting from time to time is the natural way to eat, as opposed to eating three to four times per day (Gunnars, 2017).

In other words, you've formed a habit and habits take time to change. IF's pattern is something that models the body's natural activity pattern. It calls for periods of fasting broken up by periods of eating, done in cycles. The most significant advantage IF provides is that it doesn't provide you with a list of foods to avoid or eat.

Instead, you only need to eat according to your fasting and feeding pattern, and the rest takes care of itself! There are multiple ways to practice intermittent fasting, so let's take a quick look at these.

16/8 Method

This method is also referred to as the "leangains protocol," which was developed by Swedish nutritionist Martin Berkhan. Leangains is probably the most effective IF protocol out there and reached the peak of its popularity around 2014. Unfortunately, this is when the mainstream fitness industry got wind of it, and all sorts of wrong and frankly idiotic information were peddled.

At its core, leangains are all about eating your meals within an eight-hour window and fasting for sixteen hours. Berkhan recommends adding your sleep periods to your fasting times, so if you sleep for eight hours per day, you'll be eating for eight hours, sleeping for eight and fasting awake for eight hours. It is this third period that can seem challenging.

Given this sort of a breakup, you will have to skip one of the traditionally accepted meals in society. Berkhan recommends skipping breakfast, which will probably ring alarm bells of all kinds within your head, but is the most effective way of implementing leangains (Berkhan, 2015). The method does take some getting used to and goes well beyond eating for eight and fasting for sixteen hours. You will need to train heavy as well as cycle your eating pattern based on whether you're working out that day or not. Doing this can seem a bit overwhelming, so let's take a closer look.

A Deeper Look at 16/8

There are no guidelines as to which time of the day you need to remain fasted or fed - this is entirely up to you. Losing fat is ultimately a question of how many calories you eat. As long as you eat less than you burn, you'll lose weight and gain more definition. Now, having said that, this doesn't mean you can eat whatever you want. Yes, technically, even if you do eat chocolate cake all day, and in amounts that provide less energy than what you need, you will lose weight.

However, weight loss is very different from fat loss. When losing weight, you can lose muscle as well, which is not what you want to be doing. So, yeah, sorry to say, your chocolate cake diet ain't gonna work! That doesn't mean you need to place yourself in food purgatory. Since you're fasting for as long as you are, you can get away with eating a bit more unhealthy stuff than usual. Obviously, this is not recommended, but my point is don't be worried about missing out.

Berkhan recommends three protocols based on when you choose to workout (Berkhan, 2015). And yes, you will need to work out hard and heavy. A lot of us girls have been brainwashed into thinking that if we lift heavy weights, we'll end up looking like one of those Mr. Olympia types. Another example of the utter nonsense that gets peddled. If you train like a man does, you'll look like a goddess. There, I said it.

Not because of some male-specific training regimen; it's just that when you workout with heavier loads, you're forcing your body to become stronger and put on more muscle and lose fat. In turn, this helps you look and feel younger, and you will also have more strength. Unless you choose to take steroids or hormones of any kind, you will never lose your feminine shape and body, so don't worry about that.

You can workout fasted, after one meal, or after two meals. There is no fixed number of meals you need to eat within the feeding phase. Those that workout after one meal will usually find it easier to eat just a meal with a small snack. Those who have more normal working schedules will find that working out after two meals is easier, with one meal post workout.

Meal Breakdown

With leangains, your most substantial meal should be consumed after your workout. The largest meal is defined as the one which has over 60% of your required calories. Now, word of warning, you will need to calculate your macros - that is the amount of fat, carbs, and protein you will need to eat depending on your goals with the diet (Berkhan, 2015).

The best way to do this is to use the macro calculator on Berkhan's website and calculate how much you need to eat to reach your goals. If you are overweight for your height and age, you will need to eat less than 'maintenance,' which is the number of calories you will need to eat to remain at the same weight.

Choosing to train fasted early in the morning is the fastest way to lose fat as soon as possible. However, this is also the toughest, since it calls for enormous mental strength. You will also need to supplement your diet with a lot of BCAA, which is a supplement I will cover later in the book. To be frank, fasted training gave me a lot of gains, but it was just too difficult and exhausting to implement.

The next option you have is to train after one meal. So if your eating window is between 12PM-8PM, which is what most people normally choose, you could eat your first meal, which is around 30% of the calories you need at 12 PM and then workout at 2 PM. Berkhan recommends working out no more than a couple of hours after finishing your meal.

Your post workout meal, which should be eaten within an hour of finishing your workout, can be had around 4-5PM, and this will be 60% of your calories. The remaining 10% can be eaten around 7:30 PM to finish off your feeding phase.

The last option is to workout after two meals. In this scenario, you will eat at 12 PM, then have your snack around 4-5PM or right before you get off work, and then workout after that. Your last meal, which will be the biggest meal of the day, will be post workout, and you end your feeding phase with this.

Personally, the final option of working out after two meals was what worked wonders for me. It was effortless to implement with my work schedule and other things going on. Again, you can adjust your feeding/fasting window to any time of the day to help make it easier to implement. Just don't break it up into multiple windows, which won't give you the same metabolic effect.

Workouts

Berkhan calls for heavy, full body exercises such as squats, deadlifts, bench presses, and overhead presses for maximum gain (Berkhan, 2015). These workouts will build your strength and combined with the diet regimen; it will melt the fat right off you. The biggest challenge you will find, as a woman, is doing this in a gym.

You will encounter stares from the other gym goers when they see a girl lifting heavy weights and hanging around the big dude area of the gym floor. You will feel self-conscious, but here's a secret: Those big guys staring at you are actually admiring you. The stereotype of the gym rat who goes around laughing at people is just that. More often than not, you'll find that those gym bros will walk over and give you some tips. It's their way of showing you respect.

So don't be afraid of going in there and doing what you need to do! For more in-depth and scientifically researched articles on this topic, make sure to check our Berkhan's website, https://leangains.com/. His writing style will take some getting used to, but ultimately, his website is extremely informative.

Drawbacks of 16/8

Leangains is a tough regimen to follow. While the macro calculation is pretty simple, the real test comes when you're two or three weeks into the program, and your lifts start getting heavy. There is also a temptation to complicate the program as well, and Berkhan's writing doesn't help in this regard.

While his focus is primarily on his clients, he does give a lot of information for free on his website. However, a lot of it is filled with deep scientific jargon, and he doesn't make it easy to understand what he's conveying, leaving it up to you to do further research and go down a nutritional rabbit hole.

Thus, if you hit a plateau or any difficulty, you will not find too much-personalized information. Over and above this, if you're not used to working out in a gym and have never done this before, you will find leangains and Berkhan's general tough love approach to things a bit too much to stomach.

This method is perhaps suited for those who already have some experience with IF and exercising as opposed to those who are doing this for the first time. If you're one of the latter, this will be one of those sink or swim type of situations, and it can get deeply uncomfortable at times. There are alternative approaches to IF, however, as we'll now see.

Eat Stop Eat

This program was also designed by a nutritionist, Brad Pilon, who implements IF in a different manner from how Berkhan does. Instead of fasting every single day, Pilon recommends fasting entirely at least once and up to twice per week, while regularly eating on the remaining days ("Eat Stop Eat Review (2019): A Legit Diet For Weight Loss? Or Fake Fad?", 2019).

You can choose to calculate your maintenance calorie rate with this, which will make your life easier. If not, you will need to track your weight and adjust accordingly. Either way, this is not as difficult as it sounds, and you shouldn't let this scare you away.

The underlying logic behind eat stop eat is to create a caloric deficit which will help you lose fat in a healthy manner.

Traditional methods of losing fat involve a lot of macro calculation and maintenance, which a majority of dieters don't have the mental energy or willingness to do.

By prescribing up to two days of fasting per week, Pilon takes this issue out of the equation in a precise manner. Let's look at how this works in depth.

A Deeper Look at Eat Stop Eat

Pilon recommends women eat two thousand calories per day and men eat around two thousand five hundred per day during their feeding days ("Eat Stop Eat Review (2019): A Legit Diet For Weight Loss? Or Fake Fad?", 2019). The number of fasting days per week should be at least one and a maximum of two. If you choose to fast two days per week, make sure they are not consecutive days.

When your body is in a fasted state, it will turn to any and all nutrition sources within. Thus, fat becomes a source of nutrition and will be burned as fuel. Not to mention, the fasting days give your body to the chance to cleanse itself and get rid of any unwanted toxins within it ("Eat Stop Eat Review (2019): A Legit Diet For Weight Loss? Or Fake Fad?", 2019).

The fasted state does pose a few challenges, though. Your body is liable to interpret the fasting period as being an unnatural one and is likely to start loading up on fat instead of burning it. Because fat is your body's emergency reserve for energy. Thus, your muscles will be burned in an effort to maintain your fat. The way to avoid this is to work out intensely during your feeding days.

By working out, you increase your muscle mass and communicate that this muscle should be preserved. Thus, when you fast, the body gets the message that the fasting phase is planned and that nutrition will arrive soon. After all, you wouldn't be exerting yourself hard if there was a famine going on, would you?

Thus, via the two fasting days, you end up creating a caloric deficit, up to 10% according to Pilon ("Eat Stop Eat Review (2019): A Legit Diet For Weight Loss? Or Fake Fad?", 2019), and you will lose fat. He doesn't provide any specific guidelines for what to eat and leaves it up to you to decide, as long as you hit the recommended two thousand calorie number (for a woman).

The time you wish to start your fast doesn't matter. For example, you could eat a meal at 8:30 PM and then continue your fast until 8:30 PM the following day. From a practical perspective, timing this is tough. After all, you need to nourish yourself once your fast is broken. The best way to achieve this is to start your fasting period in the afternoon and have it end on the following afternoon. This way, you've given yourself enough time to consume the required number of calories for that day.

Workouts

It is best to avoid workouts on your fasted days since you'll only be consuming water or low-calorie drinks like sparkling water. During your feeding days, it is best to perform strength training exercises, although Pilon doesn't call for as intense a workout routine as with leangains.

He does, however, prioritize strength building over cardio. Cardio is generally used to lose fat, but with your diet taking care of that already, performing only cardio will cause you to lose muscle. Thus, focus on training for strength and performing exercises in the 6-12 rep range.

If you don't know what a rep is or are wondering what exercises you should perform, don't worry, I'll cover all of this in a later chapter. For now, remember that you ought to focus on strength training and not just cardio.

You can exercise three to four days per week and follow one of the recommended workout programs which I've listed later in this book.

Drawbacks of Eat Stop Eat

While providing a more straightforward template to follow, Eat Stop Eat is more challenging to put into practice at the end of the day. The biggest reason for this is the constant weight tracking you need to do and the possibility of overeating when you come out of your fast.

The fasting period is far more drastic as compared to leangains, and this will tempt a lot of people to overeat. Not to mention, the difficulty of tracking calories before and after you break your fast. The method is a bit unclear about this, and Pilon seems to suggest that the calories will even out over time, thanks to the deficit building up.

Since this is an IF method, there is no specific nutritional guide, and the primary source of information is Pilon's book, *Eat Stop Eat*. Overall, this is a very effective method if you can manage to implement it, and the results it provides are very real. By relying on basic IF principles, and by delivering a simple template, the method is well worth a shot.

5:2

The last intermittent fasting protocol is the most beginner friendly and is the easiest to follow and understand. Title 5:2, the diet calls for eating what you want for five days of the week and on two days, eating just five hundred calories. The intention is to create a caloric deficit via the two fasting days, which are supposed to be non-consecutive (Bjarnadottir, 2018).

There are no other calorie restrictions with this diet, and it is essentially a simplification of the previous two methods. Eat Stop Eat has become the most popular type of intermittent fasting protocol right now, and the reason for this is the minimal change that is required to implement it.

By not having to calculate a lot of macros or even calories, you're free to eat as you've been doing this far. It kicks in only on the two days you have to fast and restrict yourself to five hundred calories. Over and above this, you can follow your chosen regimen of exercise, which will boost your fat loss as well (Bjarnadottir, 2018).

That's pretty much all there is to it, really! I don't even need an in-depth section to explain this further. There are, however, some cons of this method you need to be aware of.

Drawbacks of 5:2

Now, I mean this in the nicest way possible, but you must understand that this method is a hack. It will work for those who have a lot of weight to lose. Once you lose that excess weight, though, you will hit a plateau since the regimen isn't very structured.

The reason most people gain weight is that they don't know how to structure their diets. By removing this requirement, 5:2 writes a great elevator pitch for itself, but it falls short in the long run. Here's the thing: While sticking to a diet regimen is detail oriented and painful, it exists for a reason. You must put in the work to see the results.

Personally, I think the 5:2 seems to market itself as the method that takes out that complexity and appeals to our lazier sides. So you will see results at first, but don't expect it to work out over the long term. Its lack of any complexity is what causes it to fail.

So thus far, we've seen three IF methods with one being a bit complex, another being a little less and one having no complexity at all. Complexity is no guarantee of effectiveness, but neither is a complete lack of it. Ultimately, you need to look at which method you can implement the best in your life.

From a results standpoint, over the long term, there is no doubt that leangains provides the best results (Gunnars, 2017). The method not only cuts fat but also helps your body remain leaner for longer since it adjusts to the new regimen. The first mental block, with regards to skipping a meal, usually breakfast, requires energy to deal with, but this is repaid many times over.

Now if this were simply a book on intermittent fasting, I'd send you on your way with these words. However, the problems soon became real to me since implementing all of this is not an easy task. Now, this is where the ketogenic diet takes out all guesswork. By implementing a definite diet plan which you can follow, you boost the effectiveness of IF.

Why don't the creators of the previous IF plans do this, you might be wondering? Well, Berkhan does provide macro nutrition guidelines on his website, and even Pilon recommends a certain macro ratio. However, they don't insist on it, because they expect the people following it to use some common sense, according to them, and figure it out.

However, I aim to remove all the guesswork for you and give you a definite guide. I'm going to spend some time now talking about the ketogenic diet and how you can successfully implement it in your life.

Ketogenic Diet

The ketogenic diet has been prescribed as a method of managing both diabetes and for those suffering from seizures since the 1930s (Kubala, 2018). The diet is also known by its other moniker, LCHF, which stands for low carb, high fat. In a nutshell, this pretty much explains what Keto is all about.

The diet calls for reducing all forms of carbs down to the bare minimum and in its place, eating fat with a decent amount of protein. The keto diet has several benefits and can help with health issues ranging from obesity to diabetes. Several studies have been conducted that prove beyond a shadow of a doubt the efficacy of this diet. Here's just a small sample:

Obesity: A study conducted in 2003 placed sixty-four subjects into two groups and divided them based on their diet. One was placed on a high-fat diet, while the other was on a high carb, low-fat diet (Foster et al., 2003).

The researchers found that the group on the low carb diet lost significantly more weight than the other group, which was on a regular diet. This effect was observed at both the three and six-month mark.

In this study, the rate of attrition was high, and thus, it was not as effective over twelve months. However, at the six-month mark, there was no doubt as to which was more effective in tackling obesity.

Diabetes: In a study in 2006, Type 2 diabetes patients were randomly grouped into two groups, again differentiated based on their diets. One was on a low-fat diet while the other was on a high-fat diet.

Here's what the researchers concluded (Daly et al., 2006):

Fat loss was greater in the low-carbohydrate (LC) group (-3.55 ± 0.63, mean $\pm$ sem) vs. -0.92 ± 0.40 kg, P = 0.001) and cholesterol :

high-density lipoprotein (HDL) ratio improved (-0.48 ± 0.11 vs. -0.10 ± 0.10, P = 0.01).

However, relatively saturated fat intake was higher (13.9 ± 0.71 vs. $11.0 \pm 0.47\%$ of dietary intake, P < 0.001), although total intakes were moderate.

As you can see, along with the weight loss, levels of HDL, or good cholesterol, also improved. This study confirms why the keto diet is recommended as a means of managing Type 2 diabetes in patients.

Brain Cancer: While the keto diet is not a cure for this malignant disease, researchers observed a remarkable reduction in tumor sizes in patients. A study performed in 2007 (Zhou et al., 2007) found that tumor sizes decreased by 65% and 35% respectively, and this enhanced the survival rate as compared to the group which was on the standard diet.

Aside from this, glucose levels dropped and, as expected, ketone levels increased. The density of the tumors was far smaller as compared to the group on the regular high carb diet. The researchers postulated that the smaller tumor size could be explained by the fact that the tumors could not metabolize ketones for energy and hence shrunk.

These studies are just meant to show you how effective the keto diet is. To understand why and how this works, we need to understand an important concept: ketosis.

Ketosis

Ketosis refers to when the body starts burning fat for fuel instead of glucose. Let me back up for a second and explain the body's relationship to glucose and carbs. The body's first option for burning fuel to power you is glucose. Glucose is a sugar that is derived from burning carbs.

Thus, whenever you eat something, it is the carbs that get burned first, as a priority, and then if there's any more need for fuel, the body moves onto fat and then protein, which is just your muscles. If you remove the primary source of fuel, the body will be forced to move onto burning fat for fuel. Thus, the fat that you have stored in your body gets burned, and this is why eating fat makes you lose fat. Yes, I understand how convoluted that sentence is.

Your body doesn't just snap into a fat burning mode, though. For most of us, it is used to burning carbs, and thus when the supply is cut off, the body goes into a twilight zone sort of mode, where it doesn't know what is going on. During this time, it will not burn your fat efficiently, and when it finally gets the message that no more carbs are forthcoming, it switches over to burning fat.

The burning of fat releases a fatty acid that contains molecules called ketones. Ketones can be detected in your blood and urine, and their production is what is referred to as a state of ketosis. The objective of the Keto diet is to keep you in ketosis for as long as possible.

Eating too many carbs will throw you out of ketosis since your body will start burning glucose instead. Thus, keeping your carbs as low as possible is vital. Could you eliminate carbs completely? Sure, you could. However, the energy it takes to remove them entirely doesn't provide as much return for your time as simply minimizing them.

Keto Food

Keto emphasizes food high in protein and fat, preferably both. This means the below foods are perfectly acceptable on this diet:

- Meat (preferably lean)

- Fatty Fish

- Chicken (lean or fatty cut)

- Bacon

- Low carb veggies like lettuce, spinach, broccoli

- Eggs

- Butter

- Cheese

- Cream

- Olive oil, Seed Oil

- Nuts and Seeds

- Tofu

- Tempeh, Seitan

- The foods to avoid are the following:

- Grains

- Legumes

- Starchy Vegetables like carrots, potatoes

- Fruits

- Beans

- Sugary foods and drink

- Bread

- Pasta

- Flour products

Keto usually presents a problem for those who are used to consuming a lot of bread or flour-based products such as pasta. For most Americans, in other words, it is quite a change that requires planning. However, with the right preparation, which I will show you, you can easily implement this in your life.

Another point to note is that while red meat is perfectly fine on this diet, it is still wise to minimize it and stick to the leaner cuts, red meat contains a lot of saturated fat. Saturated fat is a tricky beast on which there isn't a lot of conclusive research.

Here's what we know: Excess levels of saturated fat cause cancer and other malignant diseases (Gunnars, 2017). However, some degree of saturated fat is required to possess good health. Thus, the best we can say at this point is to simply minimize it, but don't eliminate it. Practically speaking, this would mean eating red meat once or maybe twice per week, relying on chicken, turkey, and fish to make up the content of your meals.

Another sticking point is the lack of fruits on the diet. Fruits contain naturally occurring sugars, which are perfectly healthy but will throw you out of ketosis and so are not allowed. Make sure you eat a lot of green leafy vegetables, and you'll get all the micronutrients and vitamins you need.

Types of Keto Diets

While the standard keto diet, or SKD, is the one which is most widely followed. Some variations serve their own purposes. For your purposes, the SKD will be more than enough, but it's still worthwhile to look at the variations in case one of them makes sense to you.

SKD or Standard Keto Diet: This is the regular diet wherein you consume around 80-100g of protein per day and keep your carbs below 30g per day. The remainder of your calories come from fat. As you can see, this entails calculating your calories, but because you'll be combining your keto diet with IF, don't worry about hitting your calorie targets or whether you should eat something or not.

What you should do, however, is get a rough idea of how much food makes up your calorie quota for the day.

HPKD- The High Protein Keto Diet is aimed at those who wish to gain muscle with cutting fat as a secondary concern. In this regimen, the amount of protein is increased to almost one gram per pound of body weight, and carbs are maintained below thirty grams. The rest of the calories are gained from fat.

CKD and TKD - The cyclical and targeted ketogenic diets are meant for those who go through extremely intense and heavy workouts. Working out and lifting weight requires the body's anaerobic facility to be high, and the keto diet tends to suppress this. Thus, with these diets, you load on carbs before working out and then aim to return to ketosis as soon as possible, post workout.

For you, the SKD combined with IF will more than do the job, as it did for me. The variations of keto are mostly for people who are very experienced and have demanding workout routines, and you ought not to worry about any of that.

Given the benefits, combining them seems like a no brainer. However, you might be worried about inheriting the difficulties of both as well.

Well, fear not, this is why I've created the next chapter, which will give you a thirty-day plan to prep for the changes you're about to make. This next chapter will help you transition into this new regimen, and all you have to do is follow it.

CHAPTER 2:

THIRTY DAY KETO PREP GUIDE

(FAMILY FRIENDLY)

So now that you know what IF and keto are about separately, it's time to put these together into a framework that you can use to lose fat quickly and in a healthy manner. The basic structure is simple enough: you need to follow an intermittent fasting protocol and eat only the foods which are permitted on the ketogenic diet. Easy peasy, right?

Well, it is as simple as that! However, a lot of people fail at this simply because they take it easy and don't prepare. If you fail to prepare, you prepare to fail! I'm not sure who said that originally, but I once heard Usain Bolt say it, and I'm willing to take his word for it.

In this chapter, I'm going to talk all about prep work. The good news is from an IF perspective; there isn't much you need to do. Keto deserves a good look, however, since you're probably not used to eating this way.

So, let's jump in!

Intermittent Fasting Prep

The first thing you need to do is to decide which protocol you wish to follow. The previous chapter gave you three to choose from, the 16/8, Eat Stop Eat, and 5:2. I'm a huge fan of the 16/8, which is the leangains technique.

Not to say that the other two are ineffective. It comes down to your personal choice. However, if you're one of those people who is sick of research and want something cut and dried, read on!

My Recommended IF Protocol

There are no surprises here - I recommend 16/8 all the way. If you are serious about it and are comfortable with digesting the lengthy nutritional treatises Berkhan writes about on his blog, I'd say go for the full leangains approach, which involves cycling your macros on your rest days. If this puts you off, don't worry. There's a simple solution.

Don't worry about cycling carbs or even working out heavy and hard as he recommends. Instead, focus on eating for eight hours and fasting for sixteen. Work out as hard as you can for as long as you can. Now, this doesn't mean you should jog in place for fifteen minutes and call it quits.

Instead, be sincere about it and definitely do some form of strength training. I've laid out a beginner strength conditioning plan for you in a later chapter, so don't worry about having to research it all by yourself. Keep it simple in terms of this protocol. Which means you don't have to worry about cycling your macros or anything of that sort.

You'll be following the keto diet anyway, so it shouldn't be much of a concern to you. Here's the important bit though: you should define your goal before you begin. Sure, your goal is to lose fat and so on and so forth. However, it is best to write down the reason you want to lose fat in the first place.

Do you want to have a sexy body? Sure! But why? What does this give you? You see, I'm trying to ask you to reflect on the real emotional reason you want to do this. Everybody has their own reasons for pursuing things in their life, and the more you are in touch with the real reason, the better you'll push yourself through the pain period.

Make no mistake, IF combined with keto, takes work. It's my job to prepare you for what lies ahead, and I'm not going to sugarcoat it for you. To be able to make it to the other side and condition your mind and body, you need a really good reason which will push you through and get you off your backside, up and running.

Once you have your reasons down, it's time to fix your fasting and feeding intervals. The interval that works for most people is to eat between 12-12:30 PM and 8-8:30 PM. Assuming you go to bed at 10 PM and wake up at 6 AM, this means you will be skipping breakfast.

If you don't wish to skip breakfast, you'll be skipping dinner. Neither of these options is socially too friendly, but given that people usually don't meet each other over breakfast, it is socially more palatable to skip breakfast. If you have a family, this will take some explaining, but be firm and stick to your resolutions.

I'll talk about this in more detail, but you really want to recruit some additional help for the first week. If you have a spouse or significant other and if the two of you have kids, then you will definitely need help. This is because your body has been conditioned to eat soon after waking up, and during the first week, it will scream in protest at the new order of things. Keto brings its challenges, so be prepared and get some help.

If you live alone, you probably won't need additional help, and it's nothing you cannot manage. It's just that kids and a family need extra attention, which is why I recommended it. The best time to implement the new IF plus keto regimen is over the weekend. If done right, by the time Monday rolls around you'll have adjusted to the keto and your morning hunger pangs will have significantly subsided. You'll also have gotten rid of your crankiness over the weekend.

So once you've circled the date, it's time to calculate your macros! As recommended in the previous chapter, use the calculator on Berkhan's website or simply Google "leangains macro calculator." Remember, you will need to be in a caloric deficit since your goal is to lose weight. In other words, you will be eating less than what you need to maintain your current weight.

Now here's the tricky bit. Every calculator out there requires an input with regards to your activity level. The levels range from sedentary to extremely active. For the most part, you will fall between sedentary to moderately active. Unless you're a pro athlete of some sort (in which case you don't need this book) or work in construction all day long, you're not going to be highly active.

A good rule of thumb is to estimate what you think your activity level is, and then choose the level below it. This way, you're playing it safe and won't need to change things down the road. Once you input all your numbers, that's it! You will receive a number that represents your daily maintenance number.

This number represents how many calories you need to eat in order to maintain your current weight. Since you want to lose weight, subtract 25% from this number (in other words, calculate 75% of this number), and that is the number of calories you need to eat every day, within your eight-hour window.

Plan to have at least three meals. If you're not comfortable eating large meals or embarrassed by it, which is a common girl problem, then break it down into smaller meals and eat every couple hours or so. Remember to eat 60% of your calories after your workout.

When Should I Work Out?

Work out whenever you damn well, please. As much as possible, avoid working out fasted. I know I said this is the quickest way to lose fat in the previous chapter, but you'll recall I also said it's mentally exhausting. Try playing around with this once you've built up some experience. For now, make sure you work out only after eating your first meal, at the very least.

If you're used to getting up in the morning to go jogging, I'd advise shelving those plans for now. Try to reschedule your workout for another time of the day. A lot of the time, I've noticed women will do anything to avoid going to the gym for fear of being laughed at. I'm telling you, once again, that there's nothing to be afraid of. So be brave and do this!

From an IF perspective, this is really all you need to prep for. The keto side of things requires more work, but don't worry. It's nothing you can't handle!

Keto Prep

Keto prep mostly involves getting your kitchen in order and stocking up on the right stuff in your home. In short, make it as easy as you can for you to follow the diet and do not give your brain any excuses to duck out of this. You'll be surprised at how much of a genius your brain can be when it comes to shirking responsibilities.

Let's take this step by step and being with your pots and pans.

Utensils and Kitchen Equipment

If you want to make life easy for yourself, get yourself an oven. More than anything else, it is the oven which will save you a ton of time and headache over what to cook and what not to. Most homes come equipped with one these days and if not, consider buying an external one. I'm not talking about those microwave/oven/grill posers, but the real things.

Next, get yourself some baking pans and ramekins. Ramekins are those little cups you bake with in order to make small pies and tarts. You'll be breaking a lot of eggs into these bad boys, so get yourself some good quality ones.

You don't need too many baking pans - a medium and a large one will do. See if you can get a bread pan and double that as a baking dish. This will become clear in the next chapter, so trust me on this one.

The next two pieces of kitchen equipment you ought to have are a skillet and a grill. A grill is optional, but it gives a nice change of pace to things. A grill is also a handy substitute for an oven, although it doesn't have the same versatility. If you don't want an oven or think you can't afford one, go for a simple grill. It doesn't need to be one of those tailgating monstrosities, just a simple one. A skillet is a must have, since it'll make your life a whole lot easier.

Presumably, you already have a kitchen knife and forks, or if you're particularly adventurous, a spork (or fpoon), so I'm not going to go too much into that.

But I Hate Cooking!

Some of us love to cook, and some hate it. Well, for those who love to cook, this shouldn't pose too much of a challenge. If you are less than enthusiastic, though, you're going to have to suck it up. Also, cooking a decent meal isn't as hard as you think. After all, you're not presenting your dish for the privilege of being yelled at by Gordon Ramsay.

It's just you eating your cooking, so deal! Besides, I've outlined a full cooking game plan for you in the next chapter, which will make your life easier. Don't worry; your meals will taste delicious. It will require you to put just a little time in the kitchen and won't involve anything extraordinarily difficult.

If you don't know how to cook, well, this is the best time to learn how to boil an egg! Seriously though, if you don't know how to cook, master some basic cooking skills first and practice for a week or two before starting. You'll only sabotage yourself through a lack of preparation otherwise.

If you have a full-time job, then no matter what, you need to plan on packing your meals with you on the go. The great thing about the keto diet is that salads are ubiquitous, so you'll be spoiled for choice in this regard. A large number of keto meals boil down to grilling or baking some meat, throwing in on top of a salad and munching that. Throw some eggs or avocado on top of it to give it some variety.

Also, you'll be pleased to know that lasagna is entirely keto, so you won't have to stay away from Italian goodness if you're a fan of that cuisine. Plus, you can now totally indulge in the cheese platter after dinner. Dessert also opens up new avenues in the form of dark chocolate, and once you've eaten this, you'll wonder why you ever liked milk chocolate.

Oh yeah, whipped cream and creams of all sorts are OK now, so there's that. All in all, don't worry. There are a ton of meal choices for you to indulge in!

The Fog

We've now come to the biggest hurdle you'll need to overcome when adopting the keto diet. Termed variously as the fog or the keto haze and so on, this is a mental state that everyone experiences upon first beginning the diet. To understand why and how this happens, we need to step back a bit into the basics covered in the previous chapter.

You will recall that the keto diet works wonders thanks to a process called ketosis, which is when your body begins to burn fat as fuel instead of its preferred source, glucose. When you first start the keto diet, your body is still accustomed to burning and receiving carbs as the major source of nutrition.

Our bodies are remarkably engineered to help us survive many conditions. For every scenario, the body has a backup of some sort to help us deal and survive. When you first starve your body of carbs, it simply turns inward and starts burning up the existing stores of glucose, reasoning that more will be on its way shortly and that there's no need to panic.

Once these existing stores are burned off, the body lies in wait for more carbs to enter the system. Soon, it begins to realize that no more is forthcoming and that it needs to activate plan B. Plan B is burning the fat stores within the body and prioritizing the burning of fat since no carbs or minimal carbs are forthcoming.

Our bodies take around three to four days, at the most a week, to change over and adjust to the new regimen. During this period, your body is not yet accustomed to burning fat in the most efficient manner possible, and thus, whatever is being burned isn't providing the greatest amount of energy it can.

Thus, you will feel a significant drop in energy and will feel weaker. Mind you; this is just a feeling associated with a lack of energy. You aren't growing weak. You will experience irritation at the slightest things simply because you don't have the energy to deal with them.

For some people, the fog doesn't really ever go away because their bodies are not physically suited to the keto diet. If this happens to you, you should consult your doctor. For the rest of us, the fog subsides within a week at the most, with a couple of days being the usual fog period.

The best way to beat the fog is to decrease your consumption of carbs drastically. On average, in America, we consume around 400g of carbs per day. By cutting this to less than 30g, you will force your body into ketosis faster only because it has to; otherwise, it will starve.

It is recommended that you implement the keto diet over a weekend since you don't have to deal with your office colleagues or traffic and all the attendant nonsense it brings.

If you are a stay at home mom, though, a weekday is your best bet since you'll have the house to yourself and can carry things out in peace.

Ultimately, figure out what will work best in your life and do that.

Shopping

This is the easy bit. Load up on the keto staples below:

- Eggs

- Lean meat like beef and chicken

- Frozen shrimp

- Green vegetables

- Butter

- Dark Chocolate

- Low carb veggies like broccoli and cauliflower

- Avocado

- Canned tuna, sardines, and mackerel

- Mayonnaise (natural and full fat)

- Mozzarella, Parmesan, and Ricotta cheese

- Olive or nut oil like coconut, almond, etc.

- Coconut flour

- Spices

You could also opt for indulgences like the following:

- Salmon

- Fresh Tuna cuts

- Fresh Crab and Shellfish

That is all there is to shop for the keto diet. From these base ingredients, you will be able to create a wide variety of delicious dishes.

If budget is an issue, reduce your shopping staples to the following:

- Chicken breasts and thighs

- Mozzarella cheese

- Spinach and lettuce

- Mayonnaise

- Canned tuna

- Coconut oil

- Spices - spice mix, five spice mix, pepper, etc.

Restaurants

Not everyone can always eat at home all the time. It's great to go out and treat yourself. When eating out, due to the restrictions of the keto diet, you will find it difficult to dine out at ethnic restaurants that favor rice or a substitute and bread of some kind. To deal with this, you have two options.

Either you don't eat this type of food, or you make a meal here part of your cheat meal. A cheat meal is a release valve of sorts where you can allow yourself to break your diet rules. A cheat meal doesn't give you the luxury of eating how much ever you want. You can break your rules but in moderation. For example, if you want pizza, then instead of eating an entire pie, have a slice. Instead of a huge sundae, have a scoop of your favorite ice cream.

When ordering at a restaurant, stick to meat and salads, since that's pretty much what the keto diet prescribes. You can enjoy a cheesecake dessert as long as you minimize the crumble and keep in mind the number of calories present. A cheat meal doesn't give you the luxury of blowing your calorie counts out of the water. Feel free to not eat to a deficit, but don't overdo it.

The Next 30 Days

So, having finished prepping and mentally prepared yourself for the upcoming challenge, let's look at what you can expect for the next four weeks. Use this as a guide to check in and evaluate whether or not you're on the right path.

Don't expect to get everything right the first time. Everyone makes mistakes - there's no other way to learn. What matters is how you work to rectify it.

Week One

This will be your most challenging week. Hopefully, you've prepared for this as detailed in the previous sections and planned your meals out in advance. Also, be prepared for the keto fog and get ready for some low energy moments and general irritability.

It is a good idea to skip any workouts for the first few days until you've adjusted to the fog. Also, remember that your feeding window isn't something that needs to end on the dot at eight hours. If you go over by ten or fifteen minutes, this is fine. Your body doesn't measure time in such terms, so don't be a perfectionist about it.

This week is all about tracking, which is something I'll talk about in a later chapter. For now, remember to keep tracking your metrics as mentioned, and keep your carbs low.

You will feel massive cravings for bread or wheat products, and this can be a challenge to overcome. Over and above, this will be your cravings for breakfast. With the latter, you can drink some water or coffee without sugar or sweeteners of any kind to help tide you over. If it becomes a bit too much, consider sleeping later so that you don't face too much of a fasting window when you wake up.

As far as the craving for bread goes, one of the best ways to overcome this is to eat something crunchy like lettuce.

Lettuce has trace amounts of carbs, and simply chewing on this will keep your mouth occupied and your brain will quiet down. The key is to keep chewing something and not eating if you know what I mean.

Generally, by the fifth day, your fog should have disappeared entirely if it hasn't, talk to your doctor and see what they suggest. For some people, it can last as long as a week. In extremely rare cases it takes up to two weeks.

If you're not feeling a fog, then there are two possible things happening. One, your body has perfectly adjusted to the new diet, so congratulations! The second scenario is that you're eating more carbs than you imagined. Track whether your body is in ketosis (I'll cover this in the tracking chapter) and check to see if this is true if your test results are positive then great! Keep doing what you're doing.

Week Two

You should have started working out by now, and you will have certainly lost weight by this point. Note I said weight, not fat. Once you stop eating carbs, your body doesn't need to store as much water within, and this is flushed out. So expect to pee a lot more during the middle of the first week through this week.

If you are still experiencing the fog, then see your doctor. Perhaps the diet isn't for you. By this point, you should be comfortable with your fasting and feeding windows and given that you're now working out, you will begin to feel hunger pangs at night or in the morning when you skip a meal.

These are extremely challenging to deal with, and you can adopt coping strategies like drinking water or unsweetened coffee to minimize this. Keep referring back to your reason to do this and keep reminding yourself of what it is you wish to achieve by following your diet.

Keep enforcing your discipline, and it will become a muscle.

Week Three

If you've been maintaining a healthy deficit, you should be losing, at most, a pound and a half per week. So by the end of this week, you should have lost four to five pounds max. If you've lost less than this, don't worry, a pound or even half a pound per week is perfectly healthy.

If you haven't lost any weight or have put on weight, then your macro calculations are wrong, and you need to recalculate. Again, this is covered in detail in the tracking chapter.

Your calorie deficit is building up now, and your hunger pangs will be huge. This week is a turning point of sorts, where your hunger pains become more prominent than usual, but your mental ability to deal with them is also strong.

Stick to your discipline for this week, and soon, you'll be able to handle your hunger really well. It will never really go away, but you'll be able to rationalize it by thinking of hunger as fat being burned within you.

Week Four

By the end of this week, you should ideally have lost anywhere from two to six pounds of fat. If you've maintained a caloric deficit of 25% throughout, then you should expect to lose around four pounds. If you've lost more than this, then it's not just fat that has been lost, but muscle. So, recalculate your macros and start eating a bit more and keep tracking things as described in the tracking chapter.

So, there you have it! A simple four-week plan to get you losing fat in a healthy manner while gaining strength. Remember to prepare well and follow the steps outlined, and you'll be just fine.

Now, a question that usually arises is what is one supposed to eat when breaking your fast. Are there any dietary guidelines? How about cheat meals, and what's the deal with them? Well, this is what I'll cover next.

CHAPTER 3:

WHAT THE HECK DO YOU EAT WHEN BREAKING YOUR FAST?

The breaking of your fast is a crucial moment since your first meal usually sets the tone for how well you'll be able to adhere to your rules. Most people approach this meal with a pang of ravenous hunger, understandably so, and tend to gorge themselves. It is tempting to make this the biggest meal of your day, but the reality is that you need to determine the size of this meal based on your routine.

In this chapter, I'll lay out everything you need to take into consideration when breaking your fast and in designing your meals.

What to Eat and What Not to Eat

The issue of what to eat when breaking your fast is made a lot easier thanks to following the keto diet regimen. This eliminates all sorts of harmful foods like sugary and processed food (think donuts, cakes, candy, etc.). The idea is to stay in ketosis, and thanks to the fasting period, your body will be in ketosis.

The amount of hunger you will feel depends on where you are in the process of adapting to the keto diet. Earlier in the process, when your body is still not burning fat as efficiently as possible, your cravings will combine with your hunger and make you ravenous.

Later on, though, you will feel what I like to think of as keto hunger. It will be a mild and less crazed version of the carb-fueled hunger. The main thing to remember at all times is to stay hydrated. Your body will be shedding water thanks to the lower carb intake, and it's easy to lose track of how much water you're drinking.

The next thing to keep in mind is your fiber intake. We've all grown up hating veggies in some form or another, but unless you want to earn a trip to the constipation zone, you will do well to eat your green leafy veggies! Make sure you're keeping up on your intake of fiber supplements that I'll talk about in the chapter on supplements.

Now that that's out of the way let's take a look at how you can break your fast in the best way possible and in a way that causes the least intrusion.

Your First Meal

Here's the thing with the keto diet - you don't need to eat as much food in order to gain the same number of calories as with carbs. One gram of carbs releases four calories of energy, while one gram of fat released double that. Thus, a lot of people fall into the trap of feeling they're eating less and pile on more and more fat.

It's a good idea to visually train yourself by measuring out your meals and getting a feel for how much you ought to eat. It need not be accurate down to the last gram but in the ballpark. As you go on and gain more experience, you'll find that you'll start doing this automatically.

Now, the size of your first meal depends on when you've decided to work out. For those who have decided to work out fasted, this meal will be your largest, and you should consume 60% of your total calories in this meal, without a doubt. This will result in a large meal, but since you have not eaten anything since your workout, this point is non-negotiable.

For the rest, if you decide to work out immediately after the meal or after two meals, the first meal should have a healthy serving of protein and of course, fat. Make sure your protein content is high in this meal because your muscles have not been fed for a while, and your body is at a stage when it is beginning to think about possibly burning some muscle.

Preempt this by feeding it with fat and bolstering your muscles with protein.

There is a lot of sense in having a lot of protein after your workout since this is what builds muscle. However, after your workout, there is zero chance of anything you eat being diverted to create fat, and almost everything goes towards nourishing and repairing your muscles (Berkhan, 2015).

Thus, as long as your protein content in the post workout meal is at a decent level, you'll be fine. It is far more critical, therefore, to feed your muscles coming out of the fasting period. Resist the urge to overeat, which will be strong in the initial days of your fast. As time goes on, your body will learn the new feeding regimen and will adjust its hunger hormone production accordingly.

Susan, How Do I Make This Easy?

I get it. You're coming off a long period of not eating, and you're probably worried you'll go crazy and binge. Well, here's what you do. First, you whip up a large batch of keto bread and keto tortillas and keep them ready in the fridge.

Next, around an hour or so before you breaking your fast, get your protein ready. This meal could either be baked chicken breast or thighs. What I do is I keep a large batch of spicy homemade salsa ready to go. Once it's time, throw the baked chicken on the keto bread with some salsa, and you're good to go!

I have a sweet tooth, so I end the meal with a small piece of dark chocolate, and this keeps me going until my next meal, which is pretty similar calorie wise to the previous one. You can either switch it up to something else, maybe like canned tuna with mayo and then wait for your workout.

Speaking of canned tuna, it's a great option since it's high in protein, and by adding mayo and a touch of coconut or MCT oil, you get all the fat sustenance you need. Plus, it always works when you aren't in much of a mood to cook or you just plain forgot to do so.

By the way, if you're wondering what keto bread and keto tortillas are, worry not! The next section will give you the recipes for these fantastic staples. These will also go a long way towards giving your brain the impression you're eating carbs, so there's that benefit as well.

Keto Bread

- Ingredients:
- 6 large eggs
- 1/2 cup melted butter
- 1 tsp baking powder
- 2 tbsp coconut flour
- Salt

Recipe:

Place parchment paper on your loaf pan/medium baking pan. Preheat your oven to 400F.

Break the eggs into a bowl and start beating them

Gradually add the butter to the eggs. Once mixed well, slowly add the coconut flour, baking powder and salt to the mix.

Continue to beat well as the mixture thickens. If the mixture isn't thick enough to hang off your beater, then add some more flour.

Spread the mixture evenly in your loaf pan and place it in the oven.

Bake for forty minutes or until the bread is done. The best way to test for this is to insert a toothpick into the mixture. If it comes out clean, your bread is done.

Cool well and then cut into slices.

Keto Tortillas

- Ingredients:

- 4 large eggs

- 1 1/2 cup coconut milk

- 1/2 cup coconut flour

- Salt and pepper to taste

Recipe:

Break the eggs into a bowl and start beating them.

Begin making the batter by adding the coconut milk to the mix. Gradually add flour and salt and pepper. Keep beating until the consistency is to your liking.

Spread a little bit of the batter on a skillet and cook both sides until well done.

Other Alternatives

Of course, this isn't the only way to do things. You could always cook up something fancier. There are several great keto recipes out there for keto fat bombs, coconut flakes, unsweetened cacao butter and so on. As long as you make sure your meal is in line with your overall caloric requirements, it's perfectly fine.

The beauty of the IF regimen you don't need to think twice about what you're eating, as long as you hit the broad guidelines. Even if you do make mistakes, which we all do, the fasting period acts as a leveler and ensures any excess calories are burned off.

This, of course, is not a license for you to eat whatever you want, as I've mentioned previously. You still need to work out your framework. IF helps when you stray slightly over the line, not completely obliterate it.

Supplements

If you're training fasted early in the morning and maintaining a feeding window of 12:30-8 PM, then there is a bit of a gap until the first meal. It is essential that you consume the required amount of BCAA supplements as directed in the next chapter.

When breaking your fast, no matter which workout protocol you decide to follow, a protein shake is a good thing to consume since it gives you a quick boost of protein and the number of calories is also low. If you're having problems consuming less than 40% of your total calories and keeping the protein content high, add a scoop or two of protein powder.

If you're worried about what protein powder is, don't worry. I'll go over this in the next chapter.

So that's pretty much it. As you can see, there's no need to overthink the process of breaking your fast. All you need to do is align your workout schedule and your calorie consumption accordingly. Typing that previous sentence was more complicated than actually doing what it says.

Make sure you're well stocked up on your staples, and whipping up a quick and delicious meal will be a cinch!

CHAPTER 4:

HOW TO EXERCISE WHEN FASTING ON KETO
(WITHOUT KILLING YOURSELF!)

Exercise is hard, and for a good reason. If you don't put your body under some stress, you can never hope to make any progress. Exercise is also intimidating. No, I'm not talking about the gym bros and the swimsuit models that invariably seem to work out only when you choose to.

I mean that there's so much information out there that the exercise industry is just as screwed up as the diet industry is. I mean, why is it this hard to get fit? In this chapter, I'll clear all this up for you and give you a clear plan to move forward with.

Even if you don't find it to your liking, don't worry. I'll give you a framework within which you can design your workout routine and get fit in the healthiest way possible!

Exercise Basics

Before I get into the different types of workouts and timing considerations, it's necessary to step back and understand some basics. To avoid the need to repeat myself and explain terms, I'll be using and also because this stuff should be general knowledge but is presented in such a muddled manner in the mainstream media that it confuses everyone.

Generally speaking, there are two primary ways of exercising: Strength training and Cardio. Cardio stands for cardiovascular training, and cardiovascular refers to the system of the same name within you, which encompasses your lungs, heart, and a few other organs. Strength training builds your anaerobic performance, whereas cardio builds your aerobic performance.

Anaerobic refers to your ability to complete tasks without or with very little oxygen. Think of lifting something heavy off the floor. We generally hold our breath and tighten ourselves as much as possible to generate strength. Aerobic exercise refers to your performance when oxygen is available, but you need to perform the activity over longer periods.

Running, swimming, hiking, and cycling are prime examples of aerobic activity. Your performance in these tasks doesn't depend as much on your strength as it does on your heart's ability to keep pumping oxygen-rich blood over long periods of time.

Now that we've got the basic definitions out of the way let's dig deeper.

Anaerobic Exercise

Anaerobic exercise is what you see, most of the time, being performed in the gym. Which involves the lifting of weights a set number of times for a certain number of repetitions. Now, it is possible to train your cardio system using weights, but it is an inefficient use of your time. It's a bit like using a bicycle to try to win a two-wheeler race. Yes, you can technically do it, but you're probably better off trying to win on a motorbike.

When training with weights, your primary aim should be to increase your strength. Strength training helps directly build more muscle in your body, and the more muscle you have, the stronger you are. Apart from being able to lift heavier stuff, your increased muscle mass has another side effect. Your body will have less of a need to store fat.

Fat storage amounts are determined by the body using this logic. If you're weak, in case a crisis like a famine or a drought hits, you're more vulnerable to it. In other words, your chances of dying are high, and therefore, you need higher levels of emergency fuel, which is fat. If you're stronger, your body reasons that you can make it out of the crisis better, and in this case, you don't need as much fat.

That is why people who are lean can get away with eating anything they want for short periods of time. Their bodies are accustomed to converting and feeding their muscles, so by this point, it pretty much shovels everything into muscle, no matter how rubbish it might be. A great example of this was Michael Phelps back when he was winning gold medals seemingly every day.

As a part of his diet, he was consuming close to 10,000 calories per day in the form of high cholesterol, fatty, and processed food. He could get away with it because his training regimen as an Olympic swimmer demanded so much energy that his body took whatever it could get. Olympic sprinters, too, tend to consume a lot of junk food occasionally.

My point is, once you're lean, you can break more rules. However, you cannot break them for a long time and expect to get away with it. The stronger you are, that is, the more muscle you have, the better your chances of wolfing down that entire cheesecake and still having your abs show.

Strength training can be divided into three categories:

- Low rep/high weight

- Medium rep/medium weight

- High rep/low weight

Rep here stands for repetitions, that is the number of times you lift weight in a particular exercise. A set is a set of reps. So if you perform an exercise for three sets of five reps, you'll be lifting weight five times, three times each.

For strength building purposes, low rep/high weight is generally the best. That is because the weight is at its heaviest here, and you'll reach your strength limits sooner. Pushing your strength limits is a good thing because this is how you can increase your overall strength. A low rep count would be anything up to five or six reps.

Medium rep/medium weight is best for building strength and attaining a great shape. Over this rep range, a phenomenon called hypertrophy occurs, which gives your muscles excellent shape and doesn't happen with lower reps. With medium reps, you can also better isolate and work on individual muscles. A medium rep range would be anywhere from six to fifteen reps.

High reps can be used for cardio purposes. Performing full body movements like the squat or bench press for these many reps will get your heart pumping quick. However, you're better off spending your time doing cardio than high reps for this purpose. You will sometimes see bodybuilders perform high rep counts with extremely low weight, to give their muscles better aesthetics for competition. As such, you need not concern yourself with this.

So, which one should you follow? Well, if you've never worked out in a gym before, you're best off starting with low reps. I'll give you a list of exercises you can perform here shortly, so don't worry about designing a training program. Too many beginners jump into the medium rep range and don't see the results they want.

Here's the thing. To build aesthetics, you need to have a baseline of strength, which is really muscle. If you don't have this, all you're doing is toning your fat. If you skip a week at the gym, all that fat is simply going to lose its tightness and jiggle again. What you need to be doing is replacing that fat with muscle, which is what low rep ranges will do.

Exercise Program

There are several fantastic beginner strength training programs out there. The most popular one is the Starting Strength 3X5 method, which represents the sets and reps you need to perform. Another popular program is the Stronglifts 5X5 program, which is pretty much the same as Starting Strength save for the number of sets you need to perform.

Both these programs are designed the same way. They center around the back squat as the main exercise and rotate the bench press, overhead press, deadlift, and barbell row around it. You will be working out thrice a week for an hour at the most. Anything more than this is overkill, given the physical demands of these exercises.

You can find details for the programs at startingstrength.com and stronglifts.com. Both websites are excellent resources, and they give you a weekly workout plan. It's pretty simple really - you squat thrice a week and perform two out of the remaining exercises.

It is crucial that you master the correct techniques for these exercises before increasing the weight. Given that all of these movements are compound ones, in other words, you'll be using muscles from all over your body; bad form will lead to injury. So set your ego aside and learn proper form.

Here's another thing that will happen, and I might as well let you know now. You will be the only girl in your gym doing these exercises. You see, mainstream fitness advice has convinced us, women, that we need to stick to small weights and exercise bikes. Well, this is complete nonsense! Go ahead and wander over to the heavyweight area where all these exercises are usually done and stick to your routine. You'll find the more serious lifters over there will come by and give you tips and compliments - trust me.

Both the exercise programs mentioned above have certain strength standards by which you can mark your progress. Once you reach an intermediate level of strength, you can then either continue with the programs or switch to a split routine. A split refers to training different parts of your body on different days.

Generally, split routines are nowhere near as taxing as compound movements, since you're recruiting fewer muscles, but it will help target and increase strength in certain areas. With a proper split routine, you can cut down on the compound movements' frequency and find your performance on them gets better.

Bodybuilding.com is an excellent resource for split routines and to be honest, by the time you reach this level, you'll know what to look for. Aim to train for four days a week at the least, and hit all areas of your body. Incorporate one compound movement per workout. So squat one day, bench the next, followed by the overhead press on the third and deadlift on the fourth day.

One important point to note here is that before starting your strength training programs, buy yourself a good pair of flat soled shoes. Ditch the gel-filled Nikes and Asics, which are only good for running. For lifting weights, you need your feet firmly planted on the floor.

You might be wondering where cardio fits into all of this or if you should even be doing it. Well, let's look at this next.

Aerobic Exercise

It's always a good idea to perform some form of aerobic exercise after your workout. If you're used to running or swimming, though, I have some bad news for you. At this point, it is best for you to focus on building your strength. The thing with all forms of cardio is that they will build your strength up to a certain point, but not beyond that.

To perform better in your aerobic activities, you need better anaerobic performance. Think of it this way: if your body can perform anaerobically well, then it needs to divert lesser amounts of oxygen than usual to sustain it once the anaerobic activity is done. In other words, you'll be huffing and puffing less.

Keep your aerobic exercise to a maximum of fifteen minutes after your workout. Do not perform cardio before your workout, since this will deplete your strength and you will not build as much muscle as you can. It will seem odd to you at first if you're used to only performing cardio, but stick with it, and you'll soon see how much better your cardio performance gets.

So what sort of cardio should you do? Well, anything that you like, to be honest. Running, Zumba, dance classes, whatever floats your boat. The only requirement of cardio is that you need to break a sweat and move. As long as you achieve this, you'll be fine. As you begin to lift heavier weights in your strength training routine, you'll find yourself less inclined to perform cardio.

If you feel completely exhausted, don't push yourself. It's perfectly fine if you miss a day's worth of cardio and only do it twice a week. It's far more important for you to train for strength.

You will read or might have read by now that cardio is great for fat loss. Well, actually, yes it is. However, if you perform only cardio, you will hit a fat loss plateau and then stop losing more weight. The reason for this is that, as I mentioned before, cardio builds your strength up to a certain limit.

As long as your strength is being built up, you will lose fat. Once you hit this strength limit, there's no reason for your body to shed fat anymore, unless you ramp up your cardio to insane levels and force your body to burn it off.

The long and short of all this is: focus on building strength and muscle and limit your cardio to fifteen minutes post-workout.

HIIT

High-intensity interval training, or HIIT, is an alternative to cardio which has gained enormous popularity. HIIT, despite being a form of cardio, it's an anaerobic form of exercise where you push yourself to the absolute limit for a short interval and then rest for a slightly longer interval. Then, you push again, and so on for around fifteen to twenty minutes.

That's fifteen to twenty minutes without strength training, mind you. Usual steady state cardio, such as cycling or swimming, needs to be performed for close to forty-five minutes (without strength training) to have a positive effect on your fitness. With HIIT, you can cut this down in half and still reap the benefits.

So which activities can you do with HIIT? Pretty much anything! The only requirement is that you push yourself to the absolute limit. Traditional HIIT intervals are set up as one minute of work and two minutes of rest, following this pattern for fifteen or twenty minutes.

As your performance increases, you keep reducing the size of your rest intervals until you're working for a minute and resting for half a minute. A popular HIIT training method is to sprint and then walk or jog, with the sprint making up the work interval. Alternatively, you could skip rope or work the stationary bike at your gym. Swimming is not recommended for HIIT since there is the chance you could drown due to exhaustion. Neither is cycling on the road due to the dangers of traffic.

So how should you integrate HIIT into your routine, should you so choose? Well, first off, if you're doing HIIT, you don't need to perform cardio. I'm saying this because you're already doing a lot of work via strength training and you'll exhaust yourself doing things this way.

Next, don't perform HIIT after your workout. Instead, designate a separate day to do this and spend up to twenty minutes on your HIIT routine. Once you're past the beginner stage, experiment with what feels better and implement it accordingly.

So, now that you have learned the basics let's see how you can implement an exercise routine within the IF framework.

Exercise Options

As mentioned previously, you have three choices when it comes to working out. You can either work out fasted, after one meal, or at least two meals. I previously discouraged you from adopting the fasted training routine since it is incredibly taxing. However, given that it is the one which will give you the most rapid results, it's worth taking a look at.

Fasted Training

When I say fasted training, I'm going to assume you wake up early in the morning, and before getting ready for work or your household duties, you get a workout in. If, like most people, you're going to be breaking your fast around 12:30 PM, this is a problem since you will not be eating before or after your workout.

The problem with working out fasted is that you will burn muscle once your energy stores are depleted. What's more, if you don't replenish your muscles post workout, you're going to lose even more muscle mass. So all that lifting during your workout isn't worth squat.

You solve this problem via supplements, specifically BCAA supplements. BCAA stands for branch chain amino acids, and they contain the stuff that muscles and protein are literally made of. You need to take 10g BCAA 15 minutes before working out, 10g an hour after, and another 10g every two hours until you break your fast (Berkhan, 2015). That is pretty much the protocol Martin Berkhan recommends on his leangains website.

At first, you will feel odd not eating something after working out, but this is just your body reacting to your pattern up until now. Eventually, you'll find that your body will adjust to the new regimen. Just remember that the meal you break your fast with should be the largest of the day, with over 60% of your calorie intake occurring here.

Try to avoid HIIT training in a fasted state. HIIT demands an extreme amount of glycogen from your body, and performing this fasted might leave you with hypoglycemic conditions. Again, if you perform HIIT once or twice, it shouldn't be an issue. Just don't make a habit of it.

Training After One or Multiple Meals

The protocols for training after one or multiple meals are pretty much the same. You need to follow the guidelines for eating the right amount of calories per meal, with the majority of the 60% coming during your post-workout meal. Other than this, it is just a question of timing and aligning your meals with the rest of your workday.

The only time this protocol is shifted is during your rest days. That is when you will not be working out. During such days, the meal with which you break your fast should be your largest.

Which One Should I Follow?

I prefer working out towards the end of the workday and having my last meal end my feeding period. This way, I have a couple of hours or so until bedtime and am good and ready to go to sleep. There's no better sleep than the one you experience after a tough workout.

Of course, life is different for every one of us, so you should think about this long and hard. Adjusting the feeding window might be an option if you wish to avoid fasted workouts. However, if you begin eating at 7 AM, you'll have to wrap things up by 3 PM, which is a bit awkward in terms of timing.

It is a lot easier to skip breakfast than it is to skip dinner since it is psychologically difficult to go to bed on an empty stomach. I recommend the 12-8 window. Don't be afraid of supplements or think they're steroids of some kind. All supplements recommended in this book are perfectly safe and legal to consume. None of them will enhance you in any way that regular food won't.

Thus, if early morning fasted training is the only way for you to move forward, then so be it. You will need to prep additionally for the BCAA and make sure you're well stocked. I'll address the different types of protein you can consume in the supplements chapter, but for fasted workouts stick to BCAA.

There may be some of you who will be wondering whether it is OK to exercise after the feeding window closes, or late at night? Well, no. It isn't. It is imperative to feed your body with protein both before and after your workout.

If you work out at night, effectively beginning your fasting phase with a workout, you'll guarantee that muscle will burn along with fat. After a workout, muscles deteriorate thanks to the strain they've been placed under. Supplying them with protein is how they repair themselves and get stronger.

So, as you can see, depriving your body of nutrition is not a good idea post workout. With the fasted workout, you keep the deterioration at bay since you consume BCAA, which is a fast-acting protein. Then, with your first meal being the largest, you can provide whole food to your muscles. That is not the case for a late night workout.

The final factor you should consider when deciding to work out is the level of fatigue you will encounter. Initially, with both the strength training programs I've recommended, you will not feel a lot of strain. However, as time goes on, roughly around the end of the first month, those weights are going to start to feel heavy.

If you haven't checked out the programs as yet, basically, you need to keep increasing the weight you lift every workout. This way, even if you stall a few times, within three months, you'll be near an intermediate level of strength, not to mention you will look entirely different.

The negative side of this is the mental toll lifting such constantly increasing weight takes. While you'll feel great, the workouts themselves and your post workout state will be one of exhaustion. Thus, it's best to leave it for the last thing in the day, right before your final meal. This way, you ensure you get great sleep as well as go to bed on a full stomach.

The Keto Effect

Since you'll be following the keto diet while implementing the IF protocol, there are additional things you need to be aware of. First off, once you reduce your carb intake, your glycogen stores are going to be depleted. Once your body is fully adjusted to the new diet, it won't need too much glycogen to keep around as spare since it's perfectly capable of using fat now.

I mentioned in the earlier chapter that during the first week, it's best not to work out since your body will be adjusting to the new diet. By workout, I don't mean to say don't perform any physical activity whatsoever. Feel free to do some light cardio or even regular cardio.

Adopting the keto diet is going to impact your anaerobic performance, and you will find making gains in the gym difficult beyond a certain point. Furthermore, since you're on a caloric deficit, this is the worst of both worlds if your aim is to gain muscle fast. Now, there's a difference between having a goal of fat loss versus gaining muscle even though one implies the other.

If you wish to gain muscle, you need to maintain a caloric excess, which is to eat more than you need. Carbs help the muscle building process thank to the glycogen they provide. Glycogen is the body's priority as fuel due to the fact that it can burn immediately and provide instant energy.

Fat takes a bit longer to burn and thus, in situations where you need instant performance, as is the case in anaerobic activity, you will feel a drop in performance. I don't mean to say you won't be able to lift anything. It's just that you will make slower progress and will stall at certain levels faster.

Stalling refers to when your strength plateaus and you cannot go past a certain level. The way to get around this is to reduce the weight slightly and then attack the level again. Both starting strength and strong lifts go into detail with regards to handling stalls, so don't worry about this too much.

Just remember that your performance with cardio is going to be better than with strength training. That doesn't mean you should ignore strength training since your cardio is 'better.' In fact, it means the exact opposite, since by expending more energy on strength training, you'll burn more fat off your body.

Is there a way to get the best of both worlds? To have glycogen available but still follow the keto diet? Well, this is what the TKD and CKD are. However, following these diet protocols requires a lot of prep and calculation, not to mention maintenance. For anyone with a full-time job, this is akin to taking another job if you're not terribly passionate about dieting and fitness.

If this is your cup of tea, though, try experimenting with it. What you can do is consume up to fifteen grams of high GI carbs like bananas or white potatoes pre-workout, while keeping your overall carb count under thirty grams or forty. That's fifteen grams of carbs by the way, not fifteen grams of potatoes. Doing this will give you a boost headed into your workout, and you will be able to use this energy to fuel your lifts.

Just make sure your workouts are of high intensity, and then track how long it takes you to get back into ketosis via the methods I'll show you in the chapter on tracking.

So, this concludes the section on exercise. For the first time, you have some homework to do! Go ahead and check out Starting Strength or Stronglifts and understand how the routines work. They're pretty straight forward, I promise.

Once you've drawn up the routines, figure out when you can work out during your work day and how you'll need to schedule your meals, as detailed in this chapter and the prep chapter.

There will be some confusion about all of this. The next chapter will address this via a bunch of do's and don'ts you need to be aware of.

CHAPTER 5:

THE DO'S AND DON'TS
YOU MUST BE AWARE OF

If this is your first-time dieting or if you're relatively inexperienced, this whole IF plus keto thing is going to take some adjusting. Mainly because we're looking to combine two methods into a single, efficient one. Even if you have dieted before, you will recall the difficulties you had when first implementing it and the steps you had to take to overcome those difficulties.

Well, this chapter is going to serve as a primer for what to do and what not to do with everything that is going on here. It will help to check back in with this chapter to see if you're following everything correctly.

For simplicity's sake, I've divided the do's and don'ts into three sections, namely, intermittent fasting, ketogenic diet, and exercise guidelines. This way, any questions you have can be answered quickly and easily. So, without further ado, let's look at the things you need to do and those you should watch out for regarding intermittent fasting!

IF Do's and Don'ts

Let's begin with the things you should do first.

Health

Are you pregnant? Under eighteen? Are you taking prescription medicine? All or any of the above? Well, if that is the case, you should not be fasting. Always make sure to check with your doctor before making any changes to your diet. While intermittent fasting is the fastest way to get healthy and lose fat, it isn't the only way.

A good approach for you to take is to clean your diet of chemically processed food and things that are high in sugar. More than anything else, these two factors will go a long way in making sure you get healthy. Chemically processed items include things like store-bought frozen pizza, highly processed oils, and so on.

Drink water as much as possible and cut down on alcohol, and you'll be doing yourself a huge favor. Eating clean may not bring the immediate benefits that IF does, but over time, the results will show. All you need to do is stick with it.

Lifestyle

The biggest challenge you will face when adopting a new diet or fitness regimen is to fit it into your lifestyle, and it's no different with IF. Common concerns include social ones as well as mental blocks against skipping meals, etc. From a social standpoint, skipping breakfast is the easiest way to do this, but if you like hanging out late with friends and such, you will find it difficult to say no to those late night snacks.

So, make sure you have a plan of action before these events. Take into account that when you're staying up late, the hunger will seem more significant because you're awake when usually the majority of your hunger occurs when asleep.

The biggest hurdle regarding breakfast as being the most important meal of the day is technically correct if your last meal happens to be at 6 PM. If you wake up at 6 AM, that's a twelve-hour gap, and, logically, you need to eat something.

Well, with IF, your final meal is going to be a lot later than 6 PM, and there's also the fact that your body can run longer than you think without food. So stop treating yourself as a weakling and just do it!

What's Your Why?

Why are you doing this? What benefits do you expect to accrue by doing so? How will your life be better, and which goals will you reach by following through on this?

(Knowing all of this before implementing IF is crucial for your success.)

As you've seen by now, IF requires work, and that's without the keto and exercising part. Over and above, you'll be in a caloric deficit. So why are you doing this? Keep it written somewhere handy so that you can remind yourself at all times.

Moderation in Exercise

You need to train hard but know the difference between training hard and going for broke. Your body is in a stressed state, and while this is good for it, too much of it will lead to the production of cortisol. Cortisol is a hormone that is produced as part of the stress response and ultimately will lead to you gaining fat.

A rule of thumb is to leave a rep or two in the tank when working out, instead of going until failure. Going to failure on the odd set is perfectly fine, but don't do it every single time. The same goes for HIIT. Don't overdo it beyond the single day per week, and don't do it while fasted.

Supplements

Vitamins, minerals, and other supplements play an essential role in helping you with IF. During the fasted state, you will experience micronutrient loss, which you'll need to wait until the feeding period to replenish. Stock up on the necessary vitamins and make sure you're getting a good dose of them.

I'll talk about this in detail in the chapter on supplements.

Fun

Look, it doesn't have to be dreary all the time. Schedule something relaxing or fun to do during your fasted state during the weekend or if you happen to be free. Massages are my go-to secret weapon against fasted state ennui. Book yourself a session at the spa and pamper yourself. Not only will you be treating yourself, but you'll also be getting healthier while doing so!

During your downtime, steer clear of any food or hunger triggers. Don't go shopping for food when you're in the fasted state, and certainly don't watch cooking or food shows in this state. Just be smart and help yourself towards your goal!

Recruit Help

Why not talk your friend into doing this, too? If your friend isn't too keen, then sign up for forums online and join Facebook groups. There are a many of resources out there for support and help, so don't be shy to introduce yourself and get help.

Everyone struggles with new diets, so don't expect yourself to be an exception. Go ahead and recruit someone to help support you and do the same for them.

Now, here's a list of the things you should NOT do before implementing IF

Ignore Your Doctor

If you experience something out of the ordinary, according to you or anyone else, let your doctor know. If you have any doubts about all of this, then ask your doctor. If you have any questions about how some of your health conditions might be affected, ask your doctor.

You get the idea. Do not neglect to inform your doctor about what you're doing. Keep them updated and follow their advice always.

Last Supper Syndrome

You're not going to jail or the guillotine. You're just eating differently. You don't need to think of this as some sort of purgatory, all right? So, put down that cheesecake and eat as you regularly would the day before you begin your new diet.

A lot of people sabotage themselves before they even begin. Think about it: if you think of your diet as being a jail of some sort, why would you want to be in it? Why would you want to follow its rules? When was the last time you intentionally sabotaged yourself, when fully conscious?

Stop making things harder for yourself and be reasonable about all of this. It is not a big deal. You've prepared and are fully ready for it.

I'm Tough!!

A lot of us women feel the need to prove ourselves as being physically strong and competent. After all, society tells us we're weak and that the heavy lifting is what men do. Well, you need not try to be a hero and prove all the doubters wrong.

Some women take it too far by pushing too hard and too fast in the gym. Examples of this would be trying to compete with the big dude squatting next to you - except he's been doing it for years now with perfect form, and you've just begun. All you'll get out of this is a sprained knee.

This way of thinking is an insidious form of self-sabotage since it cloaks within self-improvement garb. Be on the lookout for this and follow the guidelines I've given you in this book.

Ignore Hydration

Water is the seed of life. Or something like that. You will lose water in copious amounts both during your fasted period as well as thanks to the keto regimen, so make sure to hydrate. Also, just as an aside, you don't need one of those ridiculous apps to track how much water you've been drinking all day.

You know when you're thirsty and drink when you feel so. Is your pee yellow? Drink water. Mind you, if you're going to be taking multivitamins, your pee will be yellow-tinged. A better indication is monitoring how often you need to pee. If you need to go every hour, you're probably drinking too much.

Is your head hurting? Are you feeling dizzy? Then drink some water ASAP.

Add Stress

Life can be tough. If it gets too tough, don't force yourself to go work out, which is likely to stress you out further and might push you off your diet. If you feel tired and want to sleep, go ahead and do so. Remember, the diet is more important than the workout.

If you feel tired during the workout and don't feel like you can continue, stop exercising. There's no gain in harming yourself - work within your limits. Schedule some massages and indulge in some weekend yoga to relieve your stress.

Keto Do's and Don'ts

The keto diet is a bit more challenging mentally as compared to the IF protocol since we're so used to eating carbs all the time. Added to this is the initial keto fog that everyone goes through, and you have a perfect recipe for breaking your rules. The good news is that a lot of the do's and don'ts carry over from the previous section. Thus, I'll cover the stuff that is keto specific.

Let's begin with the things you should be doing.

Whole Food

It'll be tempting to take shortcuts and eat chemically processed food that is high in fat. Avoid this temptation and clean up your diet. What I mean by this is you need to stick to real food like cheese, butter, etc. and avoid the processed stuff like marmalade and margarine.

Similarly, when it comes to meat, stick to whole lean cuts instead of minced meat, which tends to be a mixture of unwanted stuff like bone and cartilage. It's fine to buy frozen meat for cost considerations. Just stay away from pre-packaged, cooked meals that don't need refrigeration and can last for months on end.

Hydrate!

Yes, I know I've covered this, but it bears repeating. Always hydrate! Powerade doesn't count, even after the gym! Well, it will hydrate you, but you might as well drink sugar mixed with water for the good it'll do you.

Stick to good ol' water, and you'll be just fine. Follow the instructions from the previous section (Ignoring Hydration) for tips on monitoring your hydration levels. Another excellent option is to consume chicken or beef stock. Bone broth is another option which has gained popularity, but since you'll be cooking chicken and beef, the former might be better options.

Eat That Fat!

All our lives, we've been conditioned to remove fat from our diets and avoid things which are high in fat. The keto diet turns this belief on its head, and it's not going to be easy to switch overnight. You need to consciously be aware of what food you're preparing and eating.

If you don't like the marble on your meat, that's fine. However, don't subconsciously cut down on butter or cream. Stick to your portions, as per the calorie counts you did previously, and eat that quantity, this also applies equally to cooking oils. There's a lot of stuff available that are advertised as low fat and low cholesterol and so on. All the while, the healthy stuff, like olive oil and coconut oil, sits behind one of these fancy oils.

A word of caution: there is a type of oil called olive pomace oil, which you need to stay away from, as much as possible, stick to extra virgin or virgin olive oil. Extra virgin oil is what is extracted from the first cold press of the olives. Virgin is what comes on the second press.

Pomace oil is chemically extracted from the husks of the olives and is not much different from any processed oil. However, thanks to advertising standards, it is sold as olive oil and tends to be a lot cheaper than the good stuff. Stay away from this. If you want a cheaper oil, try coconut oil.

Given the high-fat quantities of these oils, you'll need less of them to cook with, so the cost will even out in the long run.

In addition to pomace oil, stay away from canola, corn, vegetable, peanut, and soy oil. A good rule of thumb is to stick to cold pressed oils. Cold pressed refers to the source of the oil being pressed to extract the oil within it. A hot press usually involves some form of chemical extraction.

Go Easy on Sweeteners

One of the drawbacks of the keto diet is the complete lack of anything sweet. Given the ban on sugar, if you have a sweet tooth, this can be a problem. Here's the good news: Once you remove sugar from your diet, you'll be amazed at how satisfied you will be with the tiniest hint of something sweet.

Even things like dark chocolate mixed with peanut butter will not taste as bitter to you. On the keto diet, you can use sweeteners but stick to the natural ones like Stevia and Erythritol. Mind you, consuming these in excess is bad as well, so you need to exercise your willpower and minimize them.

Avoid Fast Food

I mean, this is just good health advice, not keto specific. If you're going to eat clean, giving fast food, the heave-ho is a no brainer. Sometimes, you'll be pressed for time and will have to resort to it. If you do choose to go this way occasionally or for your cheat meal, then minimize the damage as much as possible.

Opt for burgers without the bun and so on. However, even the meat is of poor quality; usually, just cheap mince bound together, so it's not like there's any great nutritional value there.

Know What You're Eating

Eating something and then trying to figure out how many calories and macros you've eaten is doing things backward. Always measure your food out before you eat it and know whether or not your calorie requirements are being met.

In restaurants, this will be a problem, and no one wants to be the Karen who bores the manager with questions about the exact nutritional value of the food being cooked. Here's a simple method to follow: have as much protein as you can. Eating additional protein is not a problem. You're already avoiding the carbs, so that shouldn't be an issue.

Minimize the fat you're eating. Instead of spooning the entire cup of butter, have just half. Over time, as you get used to your portion sizes, you'll be able to estimate or feel how much is the appropriate amount. In the beginning, though, stick to protein as much as possible.

Add Seeds and Nuts

Want a quick and easy snack? Add a mixture of nuts and seeds to your diet and carry them around with you. Be careful, though. It's easy to eat too much fat with these since they're so small and you can lose track of how much you've had.

Next time you watch a movie, pack some nuts instead of starving yourself as people around you gorge themselves on popcorn.

To round things off, here's a simple don't for you:

"Sugar-Free"

I'm not going to bore you on the veracity of these labels, but generally speaking, stay away from these types of products. Just because something is labeled sugar free doesn't mean it is healthy for you. Organic is another labeling con job that occurs frequently.

The key to all of this is to stick to natural, whole food as much as possible. If you're buying eggs, buy the ones which are labeled free-range or organic (despite my previous misgivings). Stay away from the 'omega 3' eggs, similarly with vegetables and other produce.

Keto dishes are straightforward to put together since, for the most part. It's just protein with salad and a little sauce drizzled over it or cheese/butter on the side. All of that stuff is natural food and doesn't come with processed junk in it or a bunch of labels on it.

Exercise Do's and Don'ts

The lists for keto and IF overlap quite a bit so if you follow one, the other pretty much takes care of itself. But that's not the case when it comes to exercising, though. I understand that a lot of you will not have stepped foot inside a gym in your lives previously, and this fine. There's a first time for everything.

So, without further ado, here's what you should be doing in the gym.

Lack of Prep

Do you know what your workout plan is? Are you maintaining a journal with the list of exercises you need to do on that day and tracking them? Or are you deciding on the spot that you'll lift this and do that?

Remember, you need to plan things ahead of time, this will include your training routine and what it is you're going to be doing in the gym. A lot of people treat the gym as a punishment of sorts and end up walking on the treadmill while watching TV.

Don't be one of these mopes! The reason they get bored is that they haven't planned anything out or thought things through. It'll be tough at first, but make sure you plan everything about your workout, from warm-ups to finishing exercises. Speaking of warm-ups...

Always Warm Up

Not warming up is the easiest way to end up with a sprain or a pulled muscle of some sort. The best warm-ups are those that get your body temperature up but don't leave you sweating profusely and gasping for air. Walking for a few minutes at a brisk pace followed by some light yoga is a perfect warm up.

Skipping rope is also a great way to get yourself going. Another aspect of warming up is to ramp up your lifts. Warming up will not be a problem at first since you'll be lifting less weight, but as you progress, you will need to build up to your work set level. A good rule of thumb is to do five sets of warm-ups, beginning with the lowest weight and then working your way up to the weight you lifted successfully two or three workouts ago.

The aim of the ramped warm up is to let your body know that some heavyweight is coming and that it needs to get ready, this is especially true of squats. Once you've warmed up at the start of your workout, you don't need to ramp into your remaining lifts. Lift the planned weight.

Compound Your Lifts

Focus on building muscle first and then worry about sculpting your body. The best way to build muscle is to employ compound lifts like the squat, deadlift, etc. These lifts recruit almost every muscle in your body and develop what I like to think of as muscle connectivity.

In other words, your muscles learn to work with one another efficiently. So the next time you pick something up off the floor, it won't be just your back taking the load - your posterior chain and core will come to the rescue as well.

Learn Proper Form

I can't overstate this enough. Without proper form, your lifts are useless. What's more, with compound lifts, you risk major injury if you don't follow proper form. Always start with the least amount of weight and don't get caught up with endlessly increasing weight.

Remember, the goal is increased weight as long as you can maintain proper form. Learn the exercises, and if you're having problems, consider hiring a trainer to help you out with these movements. Take your time with the lower weights, and once you master them, move on to higher weight while keeping an eye out for your form.

Breaking form for a rep or two on your final set is fine, since you're pushing for higher gains and will probably be tired. You need to achieve that balance between pushing hard and relaxing your form on those tough reps and being absolutly strict to form.

Rest

Discipline is something you will need if you are to be successful. What a lot of people don't realize, however, is that in addition to doing certain things are certain times, such as pushing yourself to exercise, you also need to stay put and do nothing, like rest when you should.

In the beginning, the weight you lift is not going to be too heavy, and you'll feel as if your rest periods are unnecessary. The strength training programs I mentioned call for a rest day in between the three workout days. So, at first, you'll feel as if the rest days are not of much use and will be tempted to advance your workout.

Do not do this. True, you might not need the rest, but the reason you need to follow the routine is to build discipline. If you violate it right from the start, when the weights do get heavy, you'll set yourself up for not going to the gym at all and missing your goals. Hence, do it right from the start.

Speaking of being tired, if you feel exhausted and like you're unable to lift anything, go to the gym anyway and try to lift something. If you feel tired after this, then it's fine to skip that workout. If need be, take a week off and then get back to it. Taking breaks is a good thing, and don't let the specter of discipline throw you off course.

During your workout, make sure you take adequate rest between your sets and don't rush yourself. You need to maintain proper form, and enough rest between sets is the best way to do this.

Intensity

Make sure you maintain a good intensity with your workouts. This means take rest, but not too much rest between sets, which will result in your heart rate decreasing. However, a good intensity doesn't mean you need to be panting all the time either.

So, find your sweet spot and stay there.

Here are the things you should NOT do when it comes to training

Worry About Anyone Else

No one is looking at you or passing any judgment, so stop worrying about this. Yes, you will make mistakes, but so have all the other man mountains around you. Calm down and focus on what you need to do. Far too many women let their self-consciousness interfere with the task at hand and end up sabotaging themselves.

Don't be one of them.

Comparisons

It will be tempting when you're lifting an empty bar to look over and see the gym bros next to you pumping out squats with all the plates in the gym on his bar and wistfully wonder if you'll ever get there.

Look, comparing yourself to someone else gets you nowhere. I know this is extremely hard advice to follow in a gym, but seriously, don't do it. Practice some self-love and remind yourself of your goals regularly and how hard you're working to achieve them.

Always be kind and compassionate to yourself, and the results are sure to follow.

Doing Too Much

It will be tempting to do everything: strength training, cardio, and HIIT, all at once in an attempt to achieve maximum fat loss. Remember always to rest when you need to and keep things simple. Remember what I said about discipline above.

I Don't Want That Bulk!

Bulking has to be the most nonsensical fear that women have. I'll say it again: you will not end up looking like a dude just from lifting weights! If anything, you will look more feminine because of the way your features will be highlighted.

Unless you choose to juice up on steroids or any such unnatural thing, you will look just fine. And no, you won't end up looking like those female bodybuilders either. So relax and put your plan in action.

A Final Note

Sudden weight loss will affect your menstrual cycle, and there are some anecdotal stories of women being affected by this (Berkhan, 2015). If you maintain a healthy deficit of 500 calories per day, then you should not have any such issues. If you do have such issues, then you're probably losing too much weight too fast.

The reason for this is that your deficit is too high. Now, your deficit is made of two components: one is the amount of food you're eating, and the second is the energy you're burning. If your workouts are too strenuous, then dial it back a bit and see if it changes anything.

If your workouts aren't particularly intense and you're still losing weight, then you're just not eating enough. Increase your calorie count by 500 calories and see how that changes things. Ultimately, if nothing works, see your doctor and follow what they recommend.

CHAPTER 6:

TIPS AND TRICKS FOR MOMS

Every woman who's had kids has been there. That post-pregnancy weight refuses to budge, and you barely have any time now that you need to take care of your little one. It's a tough period for any woman and while your desire to lose weight is high, should you go ahead and implement an IF plus keto regimen?

Well, first off, it needs to be said that if you're pregnant, you should not be fasting for any reason whatsoever (Berkhan, 2015). Fasting will put both you and your baby in harm's way. As for the keto diet, it depends. Let's start by looking at this first.

Keto When Pregnant

The truth of the matter is that there isn't any conclusive research on the subject due to almost no study enrolling pregnant women out of ethical concerns. Furthermore, one of the tests your doctor will conduct is to check for ketoacidosis, which is the presence of excessive ketones in your urine and blood (Kubala, 2018).

Ketoacidosis is an extremely bad sign and will result in pregnancy complications. If you're on the keto diet, then you will be producing ketones. So how much is a good level? Well, again, it depends on your doctor. The more conservative ones will advise you to not take any chances for fear of missing harmful symptoms over regular ketones (Kubala, 2018).

Some doctors are comfortable with this, however. Indeed, some doctors even advise beginning the keto diet two to three months before you try to get pregnant since you'll be fat-adapted by the time your baby is conceived (Mullens & Dr. Andreas Eenfeldt, 2019). Doctors report reduced rates of miscarriages, preeclampsia, and morning sickness when adopting the keto diet.

What is not recommended is changing your diet once you become pregnant. Ultimately, the best thing you can do is to speak to your doctor and let them know all about your diet and lifestyle. Follow what they say, and you'll be fine. You can always lose that weight once your baby is delivered.

Different bodies run on different types of nutrition, with some resistant to carbs and some preferring fat. So, check with your doctor and follow what they recommend.

Incidentally, the keto diet has been shown to improve your chances of conceiving and improving your fertility (Mullens & Dr. Andreas Eenfeldt, 2019). So if you have problems conceiving, talk to your doctor about this and see if it works for you.

Post Pregnancy

Once your baby is born, the real issue you're going to have to deal with is whether you should continue keto or not. As mentioned earlier, intermittent fasting is out of the question since producing milk and feeding your baby will call for additional calories and you should not be reducing your food intake (Mullens & Dr. Andreas Eenfeldt, 2019).

Also, for as long as you are nursing your child, you should not be in a caloric deficit. The reasons for this are the same as that with intermittent fasting. If anything, you should be eating at maintenance or more to meet your body's needs.

So how do you go about losing fat? Well, keto is an excellent option for this, since it will induce body recomposition, which is converting your fat into muscle. It will take longer since you're not in a deficit, but this doesn't mean you should not follow it. The only thing to keep in mind is that your carb intake should be higher than on a regular keto diet, around fifty grams or more.

The reason for this is, you will lose sugar via your breast milk, and you need to replenish it to keep your baby healthy.

Case Studies

In 2015, the Swedish Medical Association published in their journal the case of a woman who suffered from severe ketoacidosis six weeks after giving birth (Mullens & Dr. Andreas Eenfeldt, 2019). She was able to recover, but doctors noted that her diet might have played a part in inducing the condition in the first place.

Ketoacidosis occurs due to prolonged periods of starvation or less than usual food intake and is exacerbated by stress and lifestyle changes. Given that the woman was following a low carb diet at the time, the stress induced by the pregnancy seems to have caused the condition in her.

She had been following the diet for a long time before giving birth, and after delivery, she suffered from symptoms of nausea, fever, and a complete lack of appetite (Mullens & Dr. Andreas Eenfeldt, 2019). Given the demands of breastfeeding her baby placed on her, it seems that she didn't eat enough food.

Now, the way this case was reported is a good illustration of how a lot of the media exaggerates and distorts basic nutritional messages. While the journal noted that the woman was following a low carb diet, the media exaggerated it as the cause of her condition, and thus created a myth (Mullens & Dr. Andreas Eenfeldt, 2019). While it's true that the low carb diet did contribute to the higher levels of ketones, thus making her more prone to ketoacidosis, it was hardly the reason for her condition.

Further examination, and indeed, the woman's statements confirm the fact that she was practically starving thanks to the lack of appetite. That being said, there is the theoretical chance of a keto diet not being compatible with breastfeeding (*Mullens & Dr. Andreas Eenfeldt, 2019*).

During the lactation process, as mentioned earlier, your body produces sugar for the milk and if you restrict your carbs too low levels, less than fifty grams per day, the stress could be too much for your body to cope with. Add to this the conditions of flu, like in the case with the Swedish woman. You can see how the low carb diet can bring about ketoacidosis.

The Swedish Medical Association reported five cases worldwide of ketoacidosis during the breastfeeding period, of which three were linked to starvation, and two were linked to low carbs (Mullens & Dr. Andreas Eenfeldt, 2019). Thus, as you can see, it's not entirely clear cut what the effect of the keto diet is on breastfeeding.

Recommended Course of Action

Dr. Andreas Eenfeldt, the founder and CEO of Diet Doctor, suggests that women can follow the keto or low carb diet while breastfeeding, but to increase their carb intake to at least fifty grams per day (Mullens & Dr. Andreas Eenfeldt, 2019). While doing this, it is also a good idea to keep an eye out for symptoms of ketoacidosis.

These include nausea, fever, and abnormal thirst. Upon experiencing any of these, you should increase your carb intake significantly, and if the symptoms still occur, then you should consult a doctor immediately.

The key, as he points out, is not so much what you eat but how much you're eating. You should be careful to provide your body with enough calories, and as long as you're providing it with enough carbs, you don't need to worry as much about the macronutrients you're consuming.

Adding fruits to your daily meals is a great way to increase your carb intake, for example. Prepare for this as soon as you can, and you'll be just fine.

Tips

It is best to get started on the diet before you get pregnant, ideally three or four months prior. Of course, not every pregnancy is planned, but this is the best scenario. Your doctor is also likely to recommend that you don't change your diet for fear of any complications so you can reap the benefits of the diet.

The next thing to keep in mind is that you should be eating at maintenance at the very least. It's a good idea to eat more than that and maintain a caloric surplus for safety's sake. Your body is going to go through the wringer soon, and you'll need all the energy you can get.

Making sure you drink enough water and eat your vitamins is a general advisory for those on keto but it applies doubly to you. Your body will shed a lot of water, and this causes a lack of micronutrients, especially electrolytes, which you need to replenish. While Gatorade and its ilk are okay occasionally, the added sugar in those drinks isn't good for the long term, as mentioned previously.

Don't keep your carb intake too low, and aim for at least fifty grams per day as mentioned previously. Also make sure you're getting enough fiber, either through food or via supplements. Keto does lead to constipation issues if you aren't getting enough fiber in your diet, so keep this in mind.

Make sure you're tracking everything, as will be explained soon in the tracking chapter. Try to maintain a journal and monitor your milk based on how many carbs you eat. You'll also be tracking your baby's measurements at this time, so as long as your child is growing at the expected rate, you're producing enough milk for them.

As always, follow your doctor's advice and keep them updated with everything that's going on. Most of all, relax and enjoy the feeling of new motherhood!

CHAPTER 7:

THE SUPPLEMENT GUIDE THAT WILL MAKE YOUR LIFE EASIER

Supplements are called as such for a reason. Your primary source of fuel should always be whole food, and you should never rely too much on supplements if you can manage it. Sometimes, this is tough. For example, if you're vegetarian, getting your quota of protein on the keto diet is going to be close to impossible.

Thus, you will need to supplement with a protein shake and BCAA. Generally speaking, I'm all in favor of protein supplements. There are, however, so many of them on the market that it makes your head spin.

In this chapter, I'm going to break down the supplements you need to have and the ones you can opt for, but they aren't all that necessary. I'll also list out the ones you don't need unless a doctor specifically recommends them. Given a large number of supplements that do exist out there, it is impossible to cover each and every one of them. If you see anything missing from here, you don't really need it in the first place.

So, let's begin by looking at the supplements you should have.

The Must Haves

The supplements in this category will help you across all three areas of the regimen, which is with intermittent fasting, the keto diet, as well as your workouts.

Protein Powder

Protein powder comes in two forms: whey and casein. Whey protein is digested and released faster, while casein is a slower releasing protein. Given that you'll be fasting, it would seem the casein is the ideal choice. However, there isn't any significant difference between the two, and you're better off sticking with whey thanks to the greater options in terms of price, as well as flavor, it provides (Van de Walle, 2018).

Since milk is not allowed on the keto diet, mix your protein powder scoops with water and add some berries (which are allowed) to the shake. Generally speaking, it's best to consume protein both before and after your workout. Given the larger size of your post workout meals, focus on consuming the bulk of your protein shake portion before your workout.

If you're on the go and happen to be busy during the time you break your fast, a few scoops of protein powder will keep you full for some time. Don't make a habit of this, however, since this is not a meal replacement.

In case you're wondering, protein powder is not a steroid of any kind, nor will it cause you to bulk up magically. It is simply protein and is no different from what you'd get eating meat. Even if you're able to meet all of your protein targets through whole food, keep some lying around the house for an emergency. Sometimes, you'll be too tired to cook, and it's important to have a ready source of protein.

Fiber

There are two kinds of fiber supplements available in the market: one in pill form and the other as powder. The opinion is divided as to whether the pills work or not. The powders, which are usually psyllium husk or flaxseed, certainly do.

I would say keep it simple and use the powder form.

Fiber is an essential part of the keto diet since the restriction on carbs results in fiber being restricted as well. A lot of dieters who begin the diet report either constipation or diarrhea, both these conditions are caused due to the higher than usual levels of protein most people are accustomed to eating.

Make it a habit of sprinkling your food with powder, they're usually tasteless and don't add anything significant in terms of calories. Be careful to stick to the recommended dosage though, or else you might find yourself pitching a tent in your toilet.

Magnesium

How would you like me to give you a superfood that regulates your immune system, gives you energy and maintains your blood sugar levels? Well, it's plain old magnesium that does this, not some exotic superfood. An ideal dosage of magnesium is in the 200 to 400 mg range (Kubala, 2018).

Due to food being heavily processed these days, the vast majority of the population suffers from a deficit of magnesium, so this isn't just a ketogenic diet thing. Additional magnesium will help you combat irritability caused by low energy, aid in muscle recovery post workout, and enable you to sleep better.

Given what you'll be going through on this regimen, magnesium is something you should have stocked. In natural food, this is found mostly in avocados, spinach, and other greens.

MCT Oil

MCT stands for medium chain triglycerides and is a form of fatty acid. MCT is mostly found in oils such as coconut oil. Coconut oil, incidentally, is one of the best sources for MCTs, so if you're cooking with this, you should be getting a steady supply of it.

MCTs are especially useful when breaking your fast because they are broken down quickly and give you an instant energy boost (Kubala, 2018). The flip side of this is the symptoms of nausea and diarrhea it can cause in some people.

Start with a small dose, half a teaspoon, and increase it gradually to see how your body adjusts.

Omega 3

The omega 3 fatty acids DPA and EHA (both of which have incredibly long spellings which you can look up yourself) are essential for suppressing inflammation and lowering the risk of heart disease (Kubala, 2018). These should be consumed no matter what if you ask me.

The richest source of omega 3 acids is fatty fish, which are a big part of the keto diet. Fish oil supplements are widely available in the form of capsules. A word of caution though - a lot of these capsules are marketed as omega 3 but actually, contain vegetable oil inside them instead of fish oil.

Vegetable oil does have omega 3 in it, but in much smaller amounts than fish oil. Make sure you purchase the real thing. Generally, look for 500 mg of EPA and 1000 mg of DHA at the very least.

Multivitamin

These supplements are a catch-all of sorts to make sure you fill in the gaps that are left from your regular diet. The most common deficiency is Vitamin D, so if you choose to supplement just that, that's fine as well.

The Good to Haves

The following supplements may or may not be of use to you depending on what you experience. Again, remember that none of these are substitutes for whole food and that you should be getting most of your nutrition from food instead of supplements.

Greens Powder

Can you absolutely not stand eating green veggies? Don't like the thought of salads? Well, then a greens powder supplement is a good alternative. There are a large number of them available on the market. A pleasant side effect of this is that you will almost certainly get your fill of micronutrients by consuming this.

Can they be used as a like for like replacement for actual greens? Well, despite containing powdered spinach and wheatgrass, you should have some green veggies with all of your meals simply because it's better to eat whole food. However, there are no adverse effects of supplementing your greens like this in the long run.

Electrolyte Supplements

During the initial stages of the keto diet, it is a good idea to keep a few packets of electrolyte powder handy in case you lose track of your fluid loss. After you adjust to the diet, you probably won't need them. The electrolytes you will need to replenish the most are sodium, potassium, and magnesium.

All of these can be found in spinach, avocado, and leafy greens. However, supplementing with this is also a good idea.

Branched Chain Amino Acids

BCAAs are vital if you choose to perform early morning fasted training. While whey and casein protein do contain BCAA, they don't carry them in the amounts necessary to make a difference (Kubala, 2018). BCAAs are released quickly into your system and thus will help prevent muscle loss when you work out fasted. This is why it's better to use these instead of protein powder, which has other nutrients and calories when fasted.

BCAAs reduce muscle fatigue and aid in recovery post workout. While you cannot substitute these for protein powder completely, thanks to the calorie count, if you're getting your protein from whole food, then consuming BCAAs right as you end your feeding period is a good idea to minimize any muscle loss that might happen.

Creatine Monohydrate

Creatine is perhaps the most researched exercise supplement in recent years. As far as aiding your workout performance, nothing beats creatine. Do you need it for a ketogenic diet or IF? Well, not really. However, if you're serious about improving your workout performance, then it's a no brainer.

As far as costs go, monohydrate is one of the cheapest versions of creatine available, and you can purchase it in various forms, as a powder, pills, or liquid. Each of these is just as effective, so you won't be losing out by choosing one over the other (Kubala, 2018).

Caffeine

Along with BCAA, this belongs in the must-haves for people who wish to carry out fasted training. Either in the form of pills or as a morning cup, coffee will get you going if you feel lethargic. A common supplement that mimics caffeine is marketed under the category "fat burner." These give you a boost of energy similar to caffeine, but without the side effects or addictive properties.

Understand that caffeine by itself doesn't burn any fat. It merely gives you a shot of energy that gets you working harder, and this is what burns calories and fat. If you're working out after meals, then there's probably no need for this. However, some people feel the need for a boost pre-workout. Incidentally, a pre-workout protein shake will give you a good boost as well, so don't think you need to rely on caffeine solely.

Probiotic Supplements

The keto diet, incidentally, is excellent for those who suffer from a leaky gut and poor digestion (Kubala, 2018). During the transition period, though, you are likely to suffer from some discomfort. Probiotic supplements will help ease this. Also, if you follow any low carb diet for a long time, your gut bacteria will die out, and you might see an increase in food allergies and such.

You can choose to either consume these in powder form or through food. The best whole food sources are anything fermented like sauerkraut or kimchi. Be careful of the added sugar in kimchi, though, and watch your carb intake with these options. The best sources of probiotic bacteria are yogurt and kefir, but these are ruled out thanks to the sugar in them. Greek yogurt is a fantastic keto option, however, and as long as you watch your carb intake, this will work well.

If you want to go the supplement way, then there are several gut health powders out there. I try to stick to whole food as much as possible, and I feel supplementing probiotics may be unnecessary.

Just remember that over the long term, you will need to add probiotics to your diet to ensure proper gut health.

Overrated Stuff

Given the popularity of keto and IF, several supplements are being marketed that, frankly, have no earthly use. They come wrapped in fancy packages with fancy names and are marketed by so-called 'authorities.'

Before you get seduced by one of these, remember that fasting has been around since ancient times. Keto has been prescribed since the early 1900s to patients. There was no need for a ton of supplements back then, and there's no need for a ton of them now.

Below is a list of stuff you don't need to worry about, not all of them are useless, mind you. Some of them are overkill for someone who's starting and are a waste of money. Supplementing these will give you fewer returns for your effort than merely cleaning up your diet and making sure you follow the guidelines listed previously.

Exogenous ketones - There's no proven research that these work.

HMB (beta- hydroxy beta- methyl butyrate) - This works, but those who lift weight at expert levels will find more use for this than beginners or intermediates.

Beta-alanine - Same as above, it prevents fatigue but nothing that a good night's rest won't cure.

Proteolytic enzymes - Seriously, just eat good food.

Molecular Hydrogen

Adaptogenic herbs - Do you like adding rosemary, basil, etc. to your food? Yes? Then you're covered.

Fat burning 'stimulants'- This is separate from fat burners mentioned above. These are marketed as somehow mobilizing your fat for better burning, whatever that means.

Binders for biotoxins - An IF supplement, these bind biotoxins together to help reduce adverse reactions during the fasted state. If that sentence made sense to you, do let me know!

Mass Monster XXXXL etc. - You've seen these products at your local GNC. While they're mostly marketed at guys, there are a few women who end up buying these thanks to their fat burning promises. Again, eat good food, and you'll be fine.

This is not a comprehensive list, of course. As I said, there are so many of these things floating around; it's impossible to cover all of them. Stick to the lists in this chapter, and you'll be fine.

CHAPTER 8:

TRACKING RESULTS AND WATCHING THAT FAT FALL **OFF!**

Tracking is the final essential element of your fat loss plan. Think of it this way: whatever you don't track, you cannot improve. You'll have to track a lot of things, from your food intake, your weight, your exercise performance and so on.

Well, I'm here to tell you that it's a lot simpler than it seems. Sure, at first you're going to feel as if you're facing a mountain of stuff, but over time, a lot of this is going to become second nature. Much like how you'll be able to approximate the calories in a meal by looking at the serving portion, you'll be able to track a lot of stuff, such as your weight, by just checking in with how you feel.

Tracking also helps you get over the dreaded fat loss plateau which every single dieter hits. There's a specific way for you to blast past this, and I'll show you how in this chapter.

So, let's dive right in and look at the things you need to track from a workout perspective!

Workout Performance

We start with the most straightforward stuff to track: your workout performance this is oddly, something you won't see a lot of gym goers do. Usually, people got to the gym and lift random stuff and go back home, wondering why they aren't making progress.

Always carry a notepad and pen with you to the gym and write down your numbers. Here's what you need to be recording.

Exercise Plan

What is your workout plan for the day? Which exercises will you be performing for how many sets and reps? What is the weight you'll be lifting? As you perform each exercise, record whether you could carry it out or not. A plan will come in handy when you begin stalling at certain weight levels and need to figure out how to move past them.

Exercise Form

Your form can be classified as a 'nice to have' to be honest. You can ask someone to take videos or pictures of you as you progress. This way you'll be able to monitor yourself for any mistakes in form or technique you might inadvertently be making. You don't need to record every single workout session. Once a week should be more than enough.

Physical Measurements

Weight

This one's obvious really. You need to measure your weight since this is the best way to make sure you're achieving progress. Now, a lot of people know how to measure their weight but go about interpreting the results in the wrong manner. Here's what you need to do.

Weigh yourself every day at the same time. So, if you weigh yourself first thing in the morning before brushing your teeth, do it at that exact moment. Don't weigh yourself the next day after having a glass of water, etc. Note down this number.

After a week, calculate the average of your measurements and note down this number. This number will be your average weight for that week. The next week, calculate the average weight. Now, compare the weekly average numbers. If the numbers are decreasing healthily, you're good. If not, you need to make some changes.

Far too many people worry about their daily weight numbers. Your weight, daily, will fluctuate for a variety of reasons either due to water retention, release, stress, and so on. If you get caught up with them, you'll be missing the forest for the trees. So take a step back and only concern yourself with the weekly numbers.

Waist Size

Here's another big one. Your weight decreasing is a good indicator of weight loss, but remember, fat loss is what we're trying to achieve. So measure your waist every day and average those numbers out. As long as you're losing inches, you're fine.

I recommend taking a loose measurement of your waist since this is a more accurate picture. Think of yourself as a tailor measuring yourself out for a new dress. Don't feed your ego and suck your belly into an extreme.

Other Measurements

If you choose to, you can measure your biceps, hips, etc. as well, but there's no benefit to these beyond a feel-good factor. If you have the time, go ahead and do so.

Pictures

Take pictures of yourself! This is going to be your before/after record, and it's vital for you to see the progress you're making visually. Stand in front of the mirror at the same spot at the same time every week and take a snap of yourself. The best time to take a picture is after you wake up.

You'll be in a fasted state, and your body is not likely to be bloated from food, so you'll get a better morale boost from these pictures.

Body Fat Percentage

Whether you need to measure your body fat percentage or not is up for debate. There's no denying that measuring it is the best way to track your progress. However, the amount of effort and money it takes to get an accurate measurement makes estimating your body fat percent a better return for your time spent.

There are several ways to measure your body fat percentage. I've listed them in order of least time consuming to most.

The U.S Navy Estimate - This estimate is good enough for the armed forces, and hopefully, it's good enough for you. You need to measure your neck and your waist along with putting your body weight and height into an online calculator. You'll then receive your body fat percent. Is this accurate? Well, it's an estimate for a reason. However, it is accurate to within a percentage point or two from personal experience.

Calipers- Measuring yourself with calipers is relatively straightforward. You pinch a fold of fat on your waist, and seven other body areas into the caliper and the resultant measurement corresponds to a particular body fat percentage. How accurate is this? Well, not very, to be frank. You can expect close to the same level of accuracy as the previous method, especially if you have a lot of fat to lose. It gets more accurate the leaner you get.

BIA Scales- Bioelectrical impedance scales send small shots of current through your body and measure the resistance encountered. Such machines are widely available, and you can carry this out in your home. Note, though, the measurements are most accurate on an empty stomach. Fluid intake significantly distorts the results.

DXA Scan- This process consists of taking two X-Ray scans of your body while you lie down. It is non-intrusive and doesn't take very long. A plus point of this is you receive information about your bone density along with details of fat concentration in your body.

Hydrostatic Weighing- File this under impractical but accurate. This method involves submerging yourself in water after exhaling as much air as possible and weighing yourself when submerged. No, don't do this in your bathtub. Hydrostatic Weighing requires specialized equipment and is usually available in research centers and don't do this at home alone.

Bod Pod- Equally impractical to everyone except professional athletes, the bod pod gives you the most accurate fat percentage based on a technique called air displacement plethysmography. Well, it's a big word, so it must be accurate!

If you can afford them, BIA scales are the best investment. As long as you're above 30% body fat, you don't need to worry too much about tracking this. Once you get below 30%, it makes more sense to track this since progress will be much tougher and you'll need to measure everything as much as possible.

Body Mass Index

Here's a twist in the tale for you. Don't bother measuring the BMI. The BMI is a simple calculation of your weight divided by your height. The resulting number is a good indicator of health. The problem with the BMI is that it isn't very accurate or reflective of health when you become lean and have more muscle mass. For instance, a lot of athletes rank as obese on the BMI standard, which is a bit ridiculous.

If you're carrying a lot of fat it is reflective, but do you need to track this? Not really, since you're tracking other numbers which give you a far better picture. The BMI is one of those mainstream numbers that get bandied about often but makes no sense.

Diet Measurements

In addition to the food prep items I mentioned in the relevant chapter, you're going to need something vital for your success: a food measuring scale. Trust me, do not skip buying one. It is essential you have this ready and know how to use it. A simple one will do - there's no need to get all fancy with it.

Food Portions

How many grams of meat are you going to cook? What about your veggies? How much oil are you pouring out?

It's going to seem like overkill at first, but the time you spend initially learning to measure quantities out is going to reap your huge rewards. By doing this at home, you'll find it easier to size up your portions in restaurants and know how much you should eat ideally.

Calorie Tracking

This one is essential, as well. There are several apps out there, with myfitnesspal being the most popular. I use a free account at fitday.com to track everything I eat. Input what you're eating throughout the day, before you eat it, and then check to see if it matches your desired calorie count.

You can also use several apps for this and program your target calorie count for the day into the app. The best thing to do is to enter everything you plan on eating for the day when your day starts. Doing this is not as difficult as it sounds since a lot of your meals will be either precooked or be derived from the same base. It'll just be a matter of adjusting one or two entries every day.

Activity Tracking

You could track the amount of energy and calories you're burning throughout the day, but frankly, measuring your body weight is just a better method, despite being slower. People got by just fine without these trackers, and I've never seen a huge need for them unless you happen to be a fitness nerd (not that there's anything wrong with that).

Keto Tracking

Ketosis Tracking

Tracking your blood or urine ketone level is essential to check whether you're in ketosis or not. This is especially the case if you've indulged in some extra carbs for your cheat meal. You should purchase urine strips, which are easily available to check for this.

These are invaluable when you first adopt the keto diet and are transitioning into it. Check for ketosis regularly and make sure you stay there. Use it to determine your ideal number of carbs. Some people cannot handle less than fifty grams simply due to biological restraints.

Ketone testing strips will solve a lot of issues for you, so go ahead and buy them.

A Sample Tracking Routine

Now that you know the various things you need to track, how do you put it all together? Well, here's a sample tracking routine for a typical day once you've adjusted to the keto diet and are regularly working out.

As you wake up in the morning, before doing anything else, you weigh yourself and note down the number. Then, you measure your waist using a measuring tape and note that down as well. If this is the seventh day of the week, then calculate the average of both numbers and compare them to the previous week.

If the number has risen, then you must have eaten more than you think the past week. Make a mental note to adjust your portion sizes down a little bit. Even better, recalculate your portion sizes based on a total caloric intake that is 250 calories less than your current intake level.

If the number is decreasing healthily, you're all good. If it's decreasing by more than 1.5 pounds per week, then you're eating far too few, and you're losing muscle as well. So, increase your intake by 250 calories in your calculations and figure out your new portion sizes.

Once this is done, you can choose to take a photo of yourself if this is the designated day. Pack your food for the day according to your schedule. If you're cooking food, then measure and cook the relevant quantities. Make sure you're carrying some nuts with you instead of snacks as you step out.

Keep track of the water you're consuming throughout the day, aiming for at least four liters of water. Before visiting the gym, make sure you have your fill of protein and consume less than sixty percent of your total calories for the day before this. Also, if you haven't already, write down which exercises you need to perform, the weight and sets and reps.

At the gym, execute your workout plan and record your numbers. If you stall, follow the stall procedure according to the strength training programs, Starting Strength or Stronglifts, as mentioned previously. Once you leave the gym, have a meal within an hour of leaving.

As the time of your feeding period draws to a close, check whether you've hit all your goals for the day. Prepare for bed and carry out the same plan the following day.

This is all there is to it: not some magic or special tasks you need to carry out. Hopefully, now you can understand why I've said that losing fat is a simple and repeatable process that anyone can follow on the IF plus keto protocol.

All this tracking has a secondary purpose, in that it will help you blast past the dreaded fat loss plateau. Let's take a look at how to overcome this.

The Fat Loss Plateau

If you've followed any diet regimen at all, you'll be aware of the fact that the fat loss plateau exists and getting past it is a significant challenge. With regular diets, this plateau occurs relatively early in the process, once the initial water weight has been shed. After a few weeks of progress, you begin to find that your weight stays the same despite continuing to do the same things.

Well, thanks to implementing intermittent fasting, you will not only lose the water weight but also not experience a plateau at all. To understand this better, we need to know why the plateau occurs in the first place. Well, if you recall from previous chapters, we saw how to lose weight, you need to be in a caloric deficit.

Now, here's an added wrinkle. Remaining in a caloric deficit is great right up until it stops working. This is because of your basal metabolic rate, or BMR, which we looked at previously, also changes as you lose fat. Your BMR reduces by almost the same amount as the percentage of body fat you lose with studies as far back as 1917 showing that a 30% reduction in calories is accompanied by a 30% reduction in BMR (Fung, 2018).

Thus, as your BMR decreases, your caloric deficit vanishes and therefore you stop losing fat. So what do you do now?

Eat even less? Well, not quite. This is harmful because the lower your BMR drops, the lower your internal body heat drops as well, and beyond a certain point, it doesn't make sense to keep cutting calories until all you're eating is a few shards of lettuce.

The key to continued fat loss is insulin. Insulin is what your body uses to extract energy from carbs. If your carb intake happens to be high, your body keeps the insulin level high and thus the body is primed to burn food that comes from outside, as opposed to looking within and burning the fat inside (Fung, 2018).

Hence, to continue losing fat, we need to keep our insulin levels low and steady. Keto and intermittent fasting are the best ways of doing this. By eating a diet that's low in carbs and fasting for an extended period, we're telling our bodies that food is not forthcoming as easily as before.

Therefore, it has no option but to look inward and start burning the fat that is within us. This is why on IF+keto, which effectively combines both insulin lowering methods, you won't encounter a fat loss plateau. The question arises, though - is it even necessary to maintain a caloric deficit to lose weight? After all, it looks like insulin is the key to everything, so why bother eating less?

Well, understand that losing fat is a two-part process comprising of what you eat and how often. Thus, the more food you eat, the greater the levels of insulin you will be producing within you. To kickstart your body into burning the fat that is stored within you, you need to eat less. Once your body gets used to the fact that nothing is going to be fed to it for sixteen hours, it adjusts and starts burning internal fat for its purposes (Fung, 2018).

Therefore, think of the caloric deficit as the initial impetus that moves your fat loss snowball down the hill. As it rolls further and further, it gets more prominent, and it sustains itself through momentum. However, a snowball can't get started without that initial force. That's what the caloric deficit is.

Focus on keeping your insulin levels low, and you'll continue to lose weight healthily. You won't need to worry about your caloric deficit after the initial few pounds you lose. IF and keto are excellent methods to keep you on track, but here are some other pointers to lower your insulin:

Avoid foods that cause energy spikes like energy drinks or too much chocolate. Dark chocolate is fine, but don't go wild with it.

Exercise regularly and engage in resistance training, which is just strength training. Hopefully, now you can see why I devoted so much time to the strength training section in this book.

Reduce stress by meditating, relaxing, and monitor your stress levels. This is because when you're stressed, your body seeks to release more energy, and this produces more insulin to mobilize whatever energy source is present (Fung, 2018).

Mental Strength

So it's 6 PM on a Friday, you're done with work, and your friends are pestering you to join them early. However, you still have a workout left, and you know that you'll have to limit your nighttime calorie intake thanks to your fast. If this sounds like a nightmare scenario to you, well, unfortunately, you're going to be facing it a lot more than you think.

Your willpower is like a muscle. The more you use it, the more it strengthens. However, like any muscle, it gets weak from overuse and a lack of rest. The key to staying the course and being mentally strong is to conserve your mental energy. This is why it is so essential for you to cut stress as much as possible and even reward yourself through cheat meals once a week.

These function as stress relievers, but again, don't run away with yourself and overdo it. Have a single piece of that brownie, instead of the entire batch. By exercising your will power during these cheat periods, you're actually building up your reserves. If you feel the need to binge or overeat, I suggest you stop dieting and take a step back.

Taking a step back seems contrary to all other advice out there, which tells you to keep pushing no matter what. Well, the reality is that you can only push for so long. Lasting change comes when you implement change in small, bite-size portions and integrate them into your life. How do you do this? Well, firstly, it's about building good habits, and secondly, it's about implementing these new habits in small steps.

If you are someone who doesn't stir off of her couch all day and watches TV all the time and considers walking to the strenuous bathroom exercise, well, no matter how hard you try, you will fail. It's not that such a person is incapable of change. It's just that the change is too big for their system to bear.

Our brains love inertia or remaining in the state they currently are in, and this is because it means processing information is easy, and there's not much stress involved. The key to implementing change is to introduce it in small, almost imperceptible steps so that your mind doesn't revolt and before it realizes it, you've installed a new habit.

Going back to our example of the terminally lazy person, the first step would be to ask herself, is walking for ten minutes a day really that bad? Probably not. So, get up and walk! Next, is reducing the TV watching time by a single show and reading a book instead that difficult? No? Well, do it then.

By repeatedly performing these actions and continually pushing as far as comfortably possible, our boundaries grow and before you know it, you'll have no trouble implementing change. If you struggle to maintain discipline, this is a symptom that the change you're trying to achieve is too much. I'm not talking about momentary feelings of laziness that hit everyone.

No, I'm talking about a constant, almost violet reaction towards something you'd like to do. If you find going to the gym excruciating, forcing yourself to go there is only going to use up your willpower, and you'll have none left to follow your diet. The key to staying strong, you see, is to use your willpower as sparingly as possible.

Another good way to motivate yourself is to inject some emotion into the proceedings.

- Why do you want to lose weight?

- Why are you doing this?

- What will it bring you?

Imagine having what you want and focus on how it feels. Focus on how good it feels and how your life changes. Even if it's a ridiculous sounding thing, it doesn't matter. This is your world! You get to imagine whatever you want.

Every day, remind yourself of why you're doing this and how it will feel when you achieve what you want. By doing this, you'll slowly and surely get there.

CONCLUSION

Intermittent fasting allied with the ketogenic diet remains the best and fastest way to lose fat and get that sexy body you've always dreamed of having. While it will seem daunting at first, remember that once you get into it and start working things out, you'll find it gets a whole lot easier.

For starters, we looked at intermittent fasting and why it's so beneficial. By narrowing your feeding window to eight hours, you're forcing your body to reduce its insulin stores whereby it begins to burn your internal body fat. A great way to kick start this process is by maintaining a caloric deficit. Although you can try to do this without a deficit, it'll take you longer and frankly, 500 calories are not as much as you think.

To boost the efficacy of this process, we add the ketogenic diet into the scheme of things. Under the rules of the keto diet, you will be restricting the amount of carbs you consume to under thirty grams or even fifty grams if that suits you better. There will be some problems when transitioning, but using the methods in this book, you'll navigate the keto fog easily. It won't always be pleasant, but hey, it won't last too long either.

Remember to always consult your doctor before starting any diet regimen. This doubly applies if you have any medical conditions or are pregnant. Even nursing mothers ought to talk to their doctors first. The best way you can reap the benefits and get rid of the eventual post-baby weight gain is to adopt the keto diet before your pregnancy. While fasting during pregnancy and the nursing period is not a good idea, the keto diet can help you immensely.

There are many pitfalls of adopting this way of eating, so make sure you review all the do's and don'ts in the appropriate chapter. Remember to relieve your stress as much as possible. This whole regimen works because it is predicated on you not harming yourself. Admittedly, it can sometimes be tough to differentiate between you being lazy and something just being entirely unsuited for you, but keep working on it and you'll be able to tell the differences easily.

Your mental state is something you should guard, and the best way to use your willpower is to use it conservatively. Which means if any situation is getting out of hand, stop, and take a few steps back. Doing this will help you reassess things and chart a better, improved course. This applies to your diet as much as the work you put in at the gym.

Do your research to determine which strength training program works best for you. It will be intimidating at first, but as I said, those gym bros respect you for venturing into their zone, given the complete lack of females in that area. So go ahead and represent!

Make sure you learn proper techniques and form before increasing the weight to prevent injury, which will be worse with compound movements. Follow a strength training routine and build your strength levels up to an intermediate standard according to the program you choose to follow. Once this is done, you can switch to a higher rep program.

Go easy on the cardio since strength training itself will take a heavy toll on you. If you choose to do HIIT, then skip the steady state cardio and do it as a separate session, instead of at the end of your workout.

Supplements will make your life a whole lot easier, but remember that whole food should be your primary fuel source. The only exception to this is protein for vegetarians and vegans, where you can substitute protein powder for all your protein needs. Again, some calorie counting is initially required to determine how much you ought to eat, but once you begin losing fat, you can maintain this level of eating.

Make sure you include lots of fiber via food and supplements in your diet, to prevent constipation, which often occurs.

Magnesium is another supplement that will help you immensely. The easiest way to get all of this is to have lots of leafy green vegetables. These are pretty low in calories, so you can have lots of them as well.

Tracking is what will make or break your results. You need to track your calories initially but can maintain your portion sizes as time goes on. Meanwhile, make sure you track your weight, waist size, and any other measurements you choose. Remember to track your progress in the gym as well to deal with stalls. Also, remember to monitor your ketone levels via test strips to figure out if you're in ketosis or not.

If you experience any symptoms of dizziness or excessive fatigue, increase the amount of food you're eating. If your symptoms persist, seek your doctor's advice.

Remember to prepare before adopting this new method of diet and exercise. It is not easy enough for you to jump in and expect to swim. It takes work, but with the right preparation and determination, you'll achieve everything you want. Remind yourself of this every time things get tough, and you feel like quitting.

Feel free to take an occasional break to clear your head. If things are getting to be too much for you, skip a few gym days instead of skipping your diet rules. However, remember to come back to your rules and keep track of your progress. Use this to motivate you and improve your life.

Finally, remember that I went through this struggle as well. I was once in your position, at a complete loss as to what to do and how to go about doing it. I certainly don't believe I'm a person blessed with anything extraordinary. All I did was take this step by step, as I've laid it out here. I guarantee that if you follow this plan, you will see results within thirty days flat!

I hope you've gained a new understanding of fat loss and dieting by reading this book. Please do let me know what you think by leaving a review!

I wish you all the best of luck and love in the world for your journey! It's going to be great girl. You got this!

SUSAN KATZ

REFERENCES

Antunes, F., Erustes, A., Costa, A., Nascimento, A., Bincoletto, C., & Ureshino, R. et al. (2018). Autophagy and intermittent fasting: the connection for cancer therapy?. Clinics, 73(Suppl 1). doi: 10.6061/clinics/2018/e814s

Berkhan, M. (2015). The Leangains Guide | Leangains. Retrieved from https://leangains.com/the-leangains-guide/

Bjarnadottir, A. (2018). The Beginner's Guide to the 5:2 Diet. Retrieved from https://www.healthline.com/nutrition/the-5-2-diet-guide

Daly, M., Paisey, R., Paisey, R., Millward, B., Eccles, C., & Williams, K. et al. (2006). Short-term effects of severe dietary carbohydrate-restriction advice in Type 2 diabetes-a randomized controlled trial. Diabetic Medicine, 23(1), 15-20. doi: 10.1111/j.1464-5491.2005.01760.x

Eat Stop Eat Review (2019): A Legit Diet For Weight Loss? Or Fake Fad?. (2019). Retrieved from http://www.healthvi.org/diet-reviews/eat-stop-eat-review/

Foster, G., Wyatt, H., Hill, J., McGuckin, B., Brill, C., & Mohammed, B. et al. (2003). A Randomized Trial of a Low-Carbohydrate Diet for Obesity. New England Journal Of Medicine, 348(21), 2082-2090. doi: 10.1056/nejmoa022207

Fung, J. (2018). Understanding Obesity. Retrieved from https://medium.com/@drjasonfung/understanding-obesity-f233fbb38dc1

Gunnars, K. (2017). Intermittent Fasting 101 — The Ultimate Beginner's Guide. Retrieved from https://www.healthline.com/nutrition/intermittent-fasting-guide#effects

Kubala, J. (2018). The 9 Best Keto Supplements. Retrieved from https://www.healthline.com/nutrition/best-keto-supplements#section7

Mullens, A., & Dr. Andreas Eenfeldt, M. (2019). Is Low Carb and Keto Safe During Pregnancy? - Diet Doctor. Retrieved from https://www.dietdoctor.com/low-carb/pregnancy

Van de Walle, G. (2018). What's the Difference Between Casein and Whey Protein?. Retrieved from https://www.healthline.com/nutrition/casein-vs-whey

Zauner, C., Schneeweiss, B., Kranz, A., Madl, C., Ratheiser, K., & Kramer, L. et al. (2000). Resting energy expenditure in short-term starvation is increased as a result of an increase in serum norepinephrine. The American Journal Of Clinical Nutrition, 71(6), 1511-1515. doi: 10.1093/ajcn/71.6.1511

Zhou, W., Mukherjee, P., Kiebish, M., Markis, W., Mantis, J., & Seyfried, T. (2007). Nutrition & Metabolism, 4(1), 5. doi: 10.1186/1743-7075-4-5

CPSIA information can be obtained
at www.ICGtesting.com
Printed in the USA
BVHW031113020819
554973BV00001B/104/P

9 781950 921133